Promise Me, Daughter

A Nurse Attorney Navigates Her Mother's Early-Onset Alzheimer's

Kathleen A. Hessler, JD, RN

Dedication

In Memory of my beloved mother,

Adele (Dale) Helen Hessler

With Gratitude
To my sister Lori, her husband John, and all my siblings

My siblings in order of birth:
Cheri, Steve, Kathleen/Kathi (me), Dan, Lori, and Sissy

Preface

This memoir chronicles my abiding love for my mother and the challenges I faced as a long-distance caregiver during her early-onset Alzheimer's. My unique background—as both a nurse and an attorney representing long-term care entities—provided me with an invaluable, insider's perspective on the operations and complexities of long-term care settings, as well as the compassionate care that is possible.

My hope in writing this book is to bring comfort and courage to those whose lives have changed because of a loved one's illness. I weave together my life, my mother's story, and the knowledge I gained while navigating her memory loss. I do not offer advice. Instead, I share educational narratives from real-life experiences to deepen understanding and foster connection. I introduce issues that families may encounter during illness.

Before describing our tender journey, I introduce my mother. She taught me the true meaning of generosity and love. Family memories and anecdotes show her deep commitment to her husband and children. Her work as a home health aide illuminates her compassion. Like many people with dementia, she lived a full and vibrant life before facing her disease.

My story, like the disease, unfolded slowly and with many pauses. Sometimes, recording facts, memories, and thoughts was therapeutic. Other times, remembering Mom's illness was too painful, and I would stop writing for long periods. My mother's course of Alzheimer's lasted twelve to fifteen years, from her first memory lapses to her death. It took a long time to find the courage to finish this book. Consequently, some timelines and details may be imperfect.

Memories fade, and while most conversations occurred in some form, dialogue is not verbatim. But I recreated them to the best of my recollection. Additionally, I kept records—photos, notes, letters, legal documents, bank statements, medical records, and government forms. These helped me recall events and activities. My focus has been to capture the emotional truth of our experience. Emotional memories often stand out more clearly in our recollections, and I was surprised by what came back to me as I wrote. I shared caregiving responsibilities with my siblings and consulted them to confirm timelines. Sometimes their memories had also faded. To protect the privacy of individuals, entities, and locations in my book, I changed some names and descriptions.

Sadly, there is still no cure for the more than seven million Americans and about fifty-five million people worldwide living with Alzheimer's or other dementias. However, researchers have made significant progress in understanding the disease and in developing targeted care measures. With the increase in awareness and available resources about the disease, care approaches are more collaborative and involve a broader community-based focus and earlier detection.

Some medications can help reduce or control symptoms. After decades of research, the U.S. Food and Drug Administration (FDA) approved two drugs for early-stage Alzheimer's disease: Leqembi in 2023 and Kisunla in 2024. These drugs have shown some promise in slowing early-stage disease. More treatments may be available in the coming years.

If you live with dementia, or are a caregiver, family member, or friend, may you find support and healing along your journey and in these pages.

Even in hardship, compassion and love can guide us.

Table of Contents

Part V
Moves and Stages

Part VI
Resolution and Reconciliation

Part I

To Promise or Not To Promise

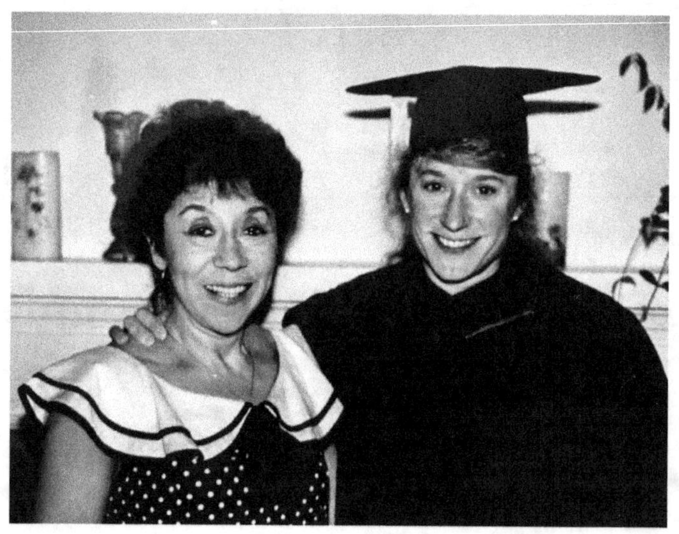

Mom and Kathleen: Law School Graduation Day, May 1991

1

Promise Me!

P romise me!
Promise me!
*Promise m*e, Kathi, that you will *never, ever,* put me in a *nursing home!"*

I still remember that devastating moment—the anguish I felt hearing Mom's pleas and witnessing the tears rolling down her cheeks. She was trying hard to hold in her sobs. We were walking back to the car on that cold January day in 1995 after an appointment with a neurologist at the University of Minnesota. He had just officially diagnosed Mom with Alzheimer's disease.

My siblings and I already knew Mom likely had early-onset Alzheimer's based on her annual physician's assessments. Her doctor told us that she had many of the symptoms of memory loss characteristic of the disease, but he was reluctant to definitively confirm the diagnosis. For more than a few years, we witnessed and discussed the distressing changes in her behavior, but we often came up with excuses for her forgetfulness.

Eight years earlier, when Dad was dying, I had some concerns about her memory, which I dismissed as caregiver stress. Additionally, Dad had asked us to watch out for Mom because he was concerned about her memory; however, her decline was not readily detectable. Even without Dad there to cover for her, it was easy to second-guess her confusion, especially since she was only fifty-two when he died.

My siblings and I had many conversations, with and without Mom, about helping her. We implemented measures to ensure her safety, allowing her to continue living in her own home. Yet, I did not want to believe the presumptive diagnosis without more proof. Despite all the observations, I continued to experience periods of denial. More importantly, I wanted Mom to visit a specialist. She needed to be treated for increasing agitation and escalating delusional episodes, and I wanted to learn about possible experimental treatments.

*****

We held hands as we approached the car. Mom was exceptionally lucid after hearing that her dementia was too advanced for any experimental medications. Despite ongoing research, there were no proven methods of delaying the symptoms of Alzheimer's, much less a cure.

Her crying was the reprieve I needed from giving a direct answer to her question about the nursing home. Her silent weeping tore at my heart. When we arrived at the car, I wrapped my arms tightly around her as she tried to muffle soft sobs. We were both well aware of the road ahead.

Mom had worked as a home health aide, providing care to people in their homes. She had cared for many patients with worsening memory loss, witnessing firsthand the progression of Alzheimer's. She saw the deterioration of a person's mind and the slow decline of the body that accompanies the disease.

She often told me stories about the men and women she cared for—how she helped them bathe and dress because they had forgotten how to button their shirt, or how to put their arms through their sleeves without prompting or guidance. On one occasion, Mom told me it was her last day caring for "a darling lady" because the daughter was placing her in a nursing home. The daughter confided that she neither had the time nor the resources to continue caring for her mom at home.

Now, I was faced with providing an honest answer to Mom, knowing much more about people suffering from memory loss and dementia than I did a year earlier. In late 1993, after working for over a decade as a registered nurse (RN), I began my new full-time career as an attorney for a long-term care company that operated nursing facilities nationwide. As the operations lawyer, I provided legal advice to the facility managers and the directors of the memory care units, which offered specialized services to residents with dementia diagnoses.

My nursing career included over seven years of direct patient care—in adult oncology research, dialysis, and pediatrics. Through these experiences, I witnessed firsthand the devastating effects illness can have on patients and their families.

We stood at the car door, silent, hugging each other. Frightened and desperate, Mom pulled back from me and searched my eyes, wanting me to promise that I would never place her in a nursing home. I drew her close again, without saying a word. Then, slowly, I withdrew to hold her gaze, her slender frame firmly in my hands.

"Mom," I said.

She continued to cry softly.

"You always told me that God never gives us more burdens than we can bear." I saw the fear in her eyes and continued to hold her.

"We will get through this, Mom," I whispered, trying to convince myself. I knew that I could not make a promise I might not be able to keep.

My mind and heart were stirring and beating, whirling like an electric mixer churning a cake batter. My soul was consumed by a mix of sadness, anger, and despair. Emotions were rapidly sifting through me, the pattern repeating.

I could only see a narrow, harrowing road ahead.

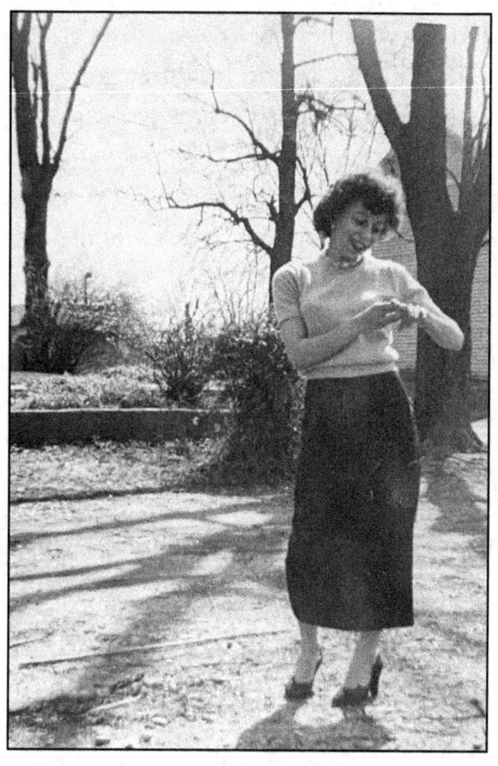

Adele admiring her engagement ring

Part II

Early Life with Mom

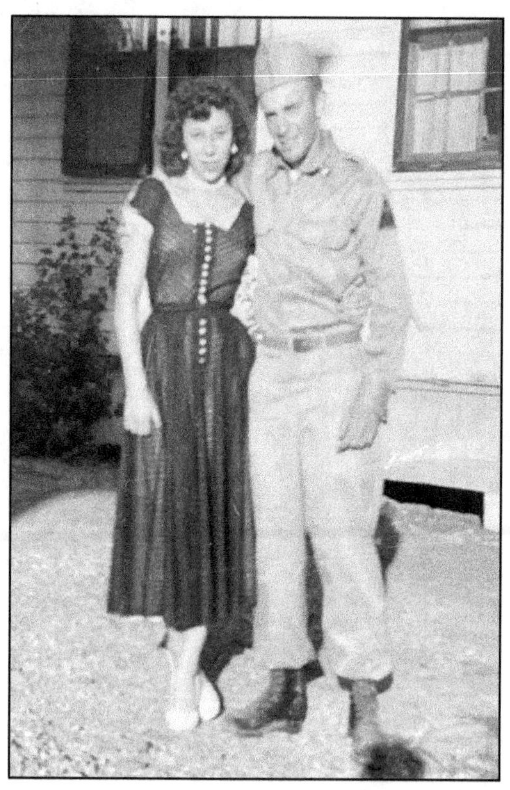

Adele and Ray circa 1953

2

Before

Smokey was barking and furiously wagging her tail as I entered the backyard from our screened breezeway. Abandoning the bone she had been chewing by the swing set, she ran toward me panting and greeting me with wet licks. I suspected she was feeling the heaviness of her bulging belly. Although not a purebred, she had the intelligence of a German Shepherd and seemed to sense the changes happening in our home.

I was twelve years old, the third of five children, and I was about to have a new brother or sister. Smokey was due the same day as Mom: May 28, 1968. The veterinarian said she would have a large, healthy litter. Mom laughed, revealing an uneasy smile when she heard the news. She was concerned about how we would manage the new litter of puppies if she were hospitalized.

As Smokey lumbered about, Mom leaned down with her knees on the cool grass and dug her hands deep into the dirt, shaping the rich soil around the tomato plants in our spacious backyard. Just as she did in our home, Mom tried to bring order to the narrow garden plot located behind the storage shed. Spring had finally arrived in St. Paul, Minnesota, and Mom was once again creating her garden.

"I love being outside," Mom said as she smiled and tilted her head up toward me as I entered the yard. I was eager for her to listen to the story I was working on for my sixth-grade creative writing class. She wanted to get the tomatoes planted before the baby arrived.

As usual, Mom stopped what she was doing when one of her children wanted attention. She twisted slowly around and sat on the ground with her legs stretched out. She placed her hands on her rounded belly and patted the thick grass beside her.

"Sit down here and read me your story," she said.

I enjoyed these moments alone with Mom. Memories of our time together and the stories she shared return to me in pieces. They are fragments of her history. I wish I had truly listened as she told the tales that shaped her life and spirit. I often study the few black-and-white photos from her childhood, including one with her Dalmatian dog. There is also a beautiful color portrait of her, with long dark curls and a radiant smile. That photo reminds me of her beauty, both inside and out.

*****

Mom married Dad when she was seventeen and he was nineteen. They met at an evening campfire event with hot dogs and s'mores. She often said she fell deeply in love with him. Since the marriage age in Minnesota was eighteen without parental consent, they drove south to Iowa in November 1952, where they were legally married after a six-month courtship.

She left school in her senior year, soon after they married, to travel with Dad while he served in the army. After basic training, he was stationed in Kentucky, where Mom joined him and gave birth to my older sister, Cheri, in November 1953.

Cheri was not yet a year old when Mom received word from her brother Alex that her mother had died suddenly. Dad was then stationed in Colorado and was unable to return for the funeral. Mom shared the painful memory of learning about her mother's death. Even years later, tears welled in her eyes as she called it "the most devastating experience" of her life.

Pregnant with my brother Steve, Mom struggled with the decision to return to Minnesota, doubting her strength to fly back alone. She feared facing the loss—especially the moment she would see her mother in the casket. After much internal searching, she found her answer in prayer. Returning to Minnesota alone, she braced herself for a rough plane ride, mirroring the mournful goodbye she was on her way to face. Hours later, as she walked wearily off the plane, her spirit rose when she was greeted by her older brothers, whose heartfelt hugs confirmed she had made the right decision.

Mom said that seeing her six siblings, relatives, and friends at the funeral provided her with comfort and a sense of peace. Still, she confided that a deep sadness dwelled within her—a pain intensified by being a new parent herself.

I cherish the black-and-white photograph of my grandmother, a plump and loving figure surrounded by her seven children. The photo rests in a gold frame on the credenza in my entryway. My mother, the youngest, was born March 8, 1935, and named Adele Helen, but was often called "Dale." After her dad died when she was eight, her oldest brother, Bill—twelve years her senior—became a stern but loving father figure. By nineteen, she was parentless.

Mom's family was poor. She felt embarrassed wearing the same two outfits every week, which her mother had purchased from the Salvation Army. Still, she attended school every day and worked diligently. When she was only ten years old, her two brothers were stationed overseas during and after World War II. At that time, Mom took on the responsibility of writing letters to them on behalf of her own mother, Helene, who could neither read nor write English. There was no question that Helene—who immigrated to the U.S. from Eastern Europe speaking only Yiddish—was greatly loved and cherished by Mom and her siblings. This was evident in the stories they told of "Ma" when they reminisced about her life.

Petite and fit—despite having delivered five children by the age of twenty-six—Mom welcomed my youngest sister on May 20, 1968, at the age of thirty-three. Just eight days later, on the predicted due date, our beloved Smokey delivered seven healthy black-and-brown puppies. Their voracious appetites added to the chaos of a house already busy with the demands of a new baby.

Moreover, I was acutely aware that Dad's drinking and entertaining at the house while Mom was in the hospital put a real strain on her.

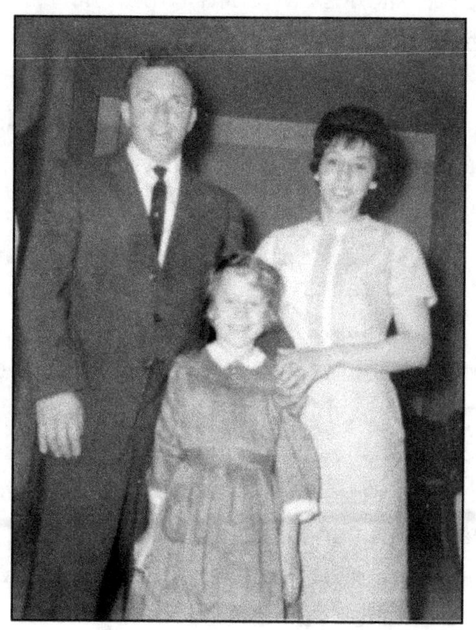

Dad, Mom, and Kathleen 1964

3

Family Memories

When I picture Mom taking time for herself, I see her walking in the neighborhood, tending her garden, or bike riding along the Mississippi River Boulevard. Later in life, she spent evenings out dancing.

Always physically active, she encouraged all her children to go outside and enjoy the fresh air, even in the cold Minnesota winters. She helped us bundle up with warm hats, colorful scarves, and sturdy winter boots before sending us out to build snowmen. She gave us carrots for the noses and raisins for the eyes. Sometimes, she came out to help us shape the snowballs and roll them on the ground to form the bottom, middle, and head of the perfect snowman. Often, we did it ourselves, but then we had to summon Mom to help us lift the large snowballs.

Barely an adult when she and Dad started their family, Mom joyfully took on the responsibilities of wife and mother. On late spring and summer afternoons or evenings throughout our elementary school years, my siblings and I played hide-and-seek, kickball, and baseball directly across our quiet street in the deep, adjoining cul-de-sac. When we saw Dad's car pull up in the driveway, we knew that within a few minutes Mom would call us to come in and wash up for dinner.

"Cheri, Stevie, Kathi, Danny, Lori! It's time for supper!" she would yell as she held open the front door, watching us kick, throw, or hit the ball with the neighborhood kids. Lori, sitting on the curb playing jacks with the other younger children, would wave to her. I loved watching Lori—who was five years younger than me—chatting with the other little girls while picking up the six-pronged metal pieces and bouncing the small ball. She was a beauty with her slender frame, long dark hair, and deep brown eyes—much like Mom's.

We came running to the inviting smells of Mom's homemade meatballs and spaghetti, freshly made lasagna, or fried chicken. I picture Mom light-footed as she moved gracefully in the kitchen, listening to the big band records of the 1940s and 1950s, or humming along to the country twang of Johnny Cash as she made dinner. Mom was happy when we were together at the table so she could wait on us; we often had to coax her to sit down to eat.

Dad owned and operated a Texaco gas station. The previous owner of the franchise had mentored and encouraged him in business, helping him purchase the station when he was in his twenties. He worked long hours repairing cars and trucks as well as running the business. Steve, Dan, Lori, and I all worked for Dad at different times in high school, either pumping gas, changing oil, or fixing cars. In my junior and senior years, I also sent out his monthly invoices.

Steve and Dan were both hard workers and helped me learn how to pump the gas and change the oil. I was sandwiched in age between the two of them: Steve, a considerate older brother, and Dan, a studious, brown-eyed jokester, always trying to lighten the mood.

In the cold and snowy St. Paul winters, Dad left the house before dawn to plow the parking lots of his business customers along Snelling Avenue. They relied on him. He was an honest mechanic and had an endearing sense of humor, drawing people to him. We knew he worked hard, and we always waited for him to come home before we sat down to dinner. This was Mom's rule.

Many times, without letting my mom know, Dad would stop at a bar on West Seventh Street in St. Paul and have a few, or many, beers. Consequently, we never had a regular dinner time. Sometimes she called the Texaco station to ask the mechanics what time Dad left for the day; she would then conjecture whether he had stopped at the bar.

From the age of seven or eight, I was on constant alert as to the level of Dad's alcohol intake. When he came home and sat on the stool by the kitchen door to take off his work boots, I stood near him to say hello. After taking in the stale smell of beer and hearing his slurred words, I would step back. If he hadn't had too much to drink, he would crack a joke with a twinkle in his blue eyes, or say, "Hey Kath, did you ace your test today?" But if he had spent hours at the bar, his eyes shone bloodshot, and the black pupils dilated. Sometimes, he stared back at me with a mean look in his eyes.

Reading his temperament, I would resolve how to behave for the evening. If I determined he was in an ill-tempered mood, I cautiously said, "Hi, Dad." Then quickly and quietly, I backed away to finish setting the table. I tried to stay away from him, or say as little as possible during dinner, after which I scrambled back up to my room, feigning the need to do homework that I had already completed.

By the time I was ten, I thought I had it down—that I had learned to respond accurately to his level of alcohol consumption to prevent conflict. I was not afraid of him when he was sober. We would play Clue as a family and watch TV while eating his famous popcorn covered in melted butter and Crisco shortening; or we would sit down to his greasy eggs and fried bologna for breakfast on Sunday.

One night, dinner had been delayed, and I was hungry. When Dad finally came home and we sat down to eat, I could hardly control my ten-year-old self. I tried. But his slurred speech was disruptive and disgusting. Dad was sitting across from me at the round table in our small dining room.

"These mashed potatoes are cold, Dale, and this meat is tough—chewy! Don't you kids agree?" His voice escalated as he looked around the table. "I should've stayed at the bar!" He started to stand up. Not wanting to argue with him, everyone remained silent. Most often, my siblings and I kept quiet when Dad was in a bad-tempered mood.

This time, I could not remain silent. I knew Mom had tried to keep the food warm while we waited for him to come home. My anger bubbled to the surface. I looked straight into Dad's angry eyes and shouted, "You are a drunk, Dad!" I was parroting what his family members called his mother. "If the food is cold, it's because we waited for you!"

He reached across the table, tipping it up to try to grab me, causing the food and drinks to slide off; I can still see the spilled milk, baked chicken, golden corn, and red potatoes on the dining room floor. He was yelling at me as I ran to my bedroom, my heart pounding while I raced up the stairs, desperate to find a place to hide—so afraid he was coming to hit me.

I had slammed my bedroom door so hard that it bounced back and hit him in the forehead as he chased after me. The bleeding wound sobered him. He packed a small bag and left the house. He did not come back for several days. After he left, Mom called me downstairs to help her clean up.

She reprimanded me, reminding me that he was my father and I needed to speak to him with respect. I did not understand this because my perception was that I was defending Mom. Why was she mad at me? While I felt relieved during his absence, Mom was sad and fretted for days. The message from her was confusing. But I learned to hold my tongue.

For years, I lived with mixed feelings of love, hate, guilt, and resentment toward Dad. I had no clear direction on how to handle these conflicting emotions, which often left me feeling lost. I remember journaling in a small, dark-green bound diary with a tiny lock and gold key. I added extra paper on which I wrote about the distressing times he came home drunk, and my feelings of anger. I taped these note papers into the journal so I could rip them up at any time. Guilt feelings followed my writing, since we were told not to share our family business with anyone. Thus, I was cautious about where I hid my diary. However, over time, I came to understand that processing and facing my emotions—no matter how conflicted I was—were critical to my growth and healing.

It was a never-ending internal battle: fighting my love for my kind, gentle, sober dad, and fearing him and worrying about us when he drank. My loyalty and fear were often at odds, and this contradiction shaped my childhood. Yet, despite the distressing times and my core conflict, we made some standout happy memories together.

Birthdays were special occasions in our home, and Dad made an effort to be on time for dinner. Every birthday was celebrated by the birthday child's favorite meal made by Mom, complete with a homemade cake. Dad's birthday was always celebrated with a large, juicy steak accompanied by sautéed mushrooms and a baked potato with lots of butter and mounds of sour cream. Most years, I chose her famous fried chicken, coated with a golden, thick batter, and accompanied by cooked corn and buttery mashed potatoes. My choice for dessert was a made-from-scratch, almond-flavored, white two-layer cake. Even as a child, I recognized the efforts Mom made to cook and bake for us.

Although it was a lot of work for Mom, every July we packed the car—with a boat and trailer in tow—and traveled four hours northwest to Detroit Lakes, Minnesota. Our suitcases and groceries were packed under a canvas cover in the modest fishing and water ski boat. Mom, always cognizant of the family budget, usually went grocery shopping before we traveled north because she said the groceries were cheaper in the Twin Cities.

Dad would stop only once at the halfway mark for gas and a bathroom break. Occasionally, to our delight, he stopped in New York Mills for ice cream. After each stretch, we rotated positions. My older sister, Cheri, cheerily moved over to make room for me by the window, and Steve gave his seat to Dan without complaint. Lori sat in the front, sandwiched between our parents. It was a tight ride in the back, but we always behaved when we were around Dad. After Sissy was born, he bought a station wagon with a rear-facing seat. I enjoyed watching the oncoming cars, delighting in the great stretches of green farmland and the inviting lakes interspersed along the way.

Dad rented a cabin for two weeks at DeSart's Resort, located on the shore of Little Floyd Lake; it was a small family-owned business with six rustic-style cabins. This became our annual family vacation and a cherished tradition. Alice and Wayne DeSart became Mom and Dad's lifelong friends. The bright pink painted exterior of the cabins and the large recreation building were as cheerful as the DeSarts' smiles and personalities.

We enjoyed seeing the same families every year. On July 20, 1969, the entire group of resort guests assembled in the recreation room and watched as Neil Armstrong made history by being the first human to walk on the moon.

Every year, we took pleasure in fishing, swimming, and water skiing. I fished alone with Dad in the early morning hours on the calm lake. He taught me how to bait my own hook and cast out into the deep waters. We sat in silence as the sun came up—our fishing lines in the lake with worms wrapped around the hooks—watching the red and white bobbers floating on top of the dark water—waiting for the sunfish and crappies to bite.

Mom did not like to fish or to eat them—except for McDonald's fish sandwiches. My siblings and I laugh when we think of the irony of enjoying fast-food fish sandwiches but not freshwater crappies, bass, or walleye. Nevertheless, Mom cooked fish dinners for her family even though she struggled with the strong smell.

Dad taught me how to cut and clean the catch for the wonderful dinners Mom prepared. After I was done filleting the bluegill sunfish or crappies in the stinky, rustic woodshed, I discarded the bones, rinsed the fleshy pieces, and took them to Mom. When making dinner, she dipped the fresh, boneless hunks into her famous beer batter coating before frying. Sometime after Dad's death, I ended up with his fillet knife, which rests in one of my kitchen drawers. Whenever I open that drawer, I am reminded of the happy times I had fishing with him.

At the lake, Mom would go down to the beach area during the day to sit and visit with the other guests. Sometimes, she sat alone and read a magazine, applying a light layer of Coppertone suntan lotion to her muscular arms and firm legs. She tanned easily with her olive skin, dark brown eyes, and thick hair that was part of her Eastern European Jewish ancestry. She would glance up from her magazine to watch us play in the water while catching a few minutes of relaxation.

Mom wore blue jeans when my friends' older parents wore polyester pants. A caring and responsible mother, she laughed easily and revealed her playful side when she was relaxed. An ardent encourager and supporter, her energy was devoted to providing for the needs of her husband, children, and household. She thrived on watching her kids grow and expand their horizons. She encouraged me to venture out into the world and approved of my plans to live and work in Europe after high school, while many of my teachers discouraged me from taking a gap year before college.

My conversations with Dad were limited during my last year of high school. I didn't share much with him. I had built up a large storehouse of anger about his drinking and my observations on how it affected Mom. She could not hide her pain from me. I believed that since I was using my own money to travel, it justified holding my plans close to my heart. In addition to the money I received as graduation presents, I had worked as a waitress in a Chinese restaurant during my last two years of high school. I also earned a fair wage for preparing and mailing the Texaco station invoices on a monthly basis. I was a good saver and was committed to being independent.

My mom noticed I was avoiding conversations with Dad. She talked to me about it and encouraged me to have a relationship with him. "You live in the same house. You need to talk with him. He's your dad," she would say. Still, I could only talk to him in passing; my anger went deep. I knew Mom still loved Dad by the affection she showed him when he was sober. I knew she was committed to staying with him, despite my pleas to her to seek a divorce. She said he was a "responsible alcoholic," providing well for our family while also expressing fear of how he would react to a divorce.

In an effort to make peace, I offered to babysit my younger siblings while they went away for occasional weekends. I thought maybe time alone together would ease Mom's tensions. I knew that I would be leaving home soon after high school.

"I will live vicariously through your adventures," Mom told me as I made my final preparations to go overseas after graduation. "Write to me about the places you see and the people you meet. Stay safe. I love you."

"Thank you, Mom. I love you too," I said. And so, I wrote often. I could visualize the smile on Mom's face when she opened my lengthy and newsy letters. It made me happy. Mom had faith in me. She never doubted that I would continue my education after my travels.

She was the person who had the most influence on me during my childhood. I cherish my vivid memories of time with her and cling to the recollections of the stories she shared, trying to diminish the sad memories of her life and of her physical and mental decline.

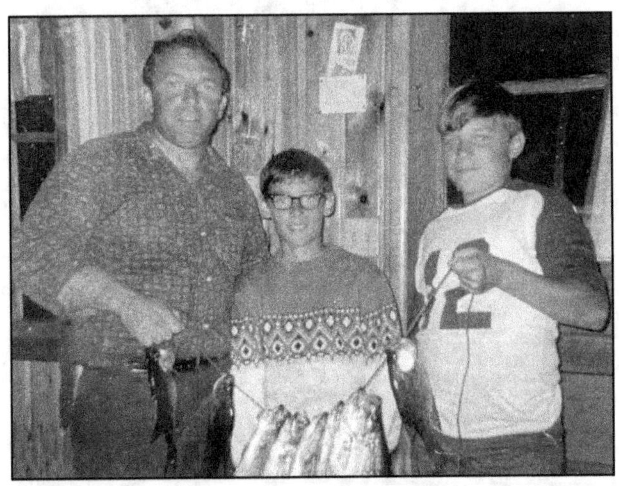

Dad and his sons, Detroit Lakes, Minnesota

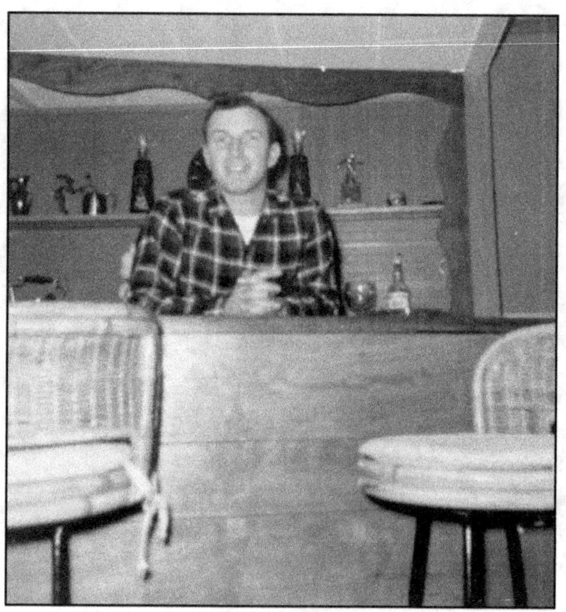

Dad, behind his bar in the recreation room

4

Sobering Choices

My heart ached, and my happiness plummeted upon returning to Minnesota in the summer of 1976. After two years away, my world had expanded, and I had grown from my experiences abroad—looking at life through a wide-open lens. Yet, the situation at home remained stagnant. My mom still agonized over my dad's drinking, a quiet despair that had put her life on hold. In retrospect, I realized that when I left for Europe on a one-way ticket in 1974, I was running away from the chaos and unpredictability in our home.

Mom maintained a good-natured exterior and still kept a spotless home, but I observed her withdraw from friends and neighbors. Her isolation grew, especially after Dad showed up drunk at a lounge when she was enjoying a rare evening out with her friends.

Thankfully, the days of escalating arguments were over. In the past, Mom would run to the yellow rotary telephone on the kitchen wall to call the police, but Dad would beat her to it, yanking out the cord to disable the phone. This destructive exercise seemed to calm him, and he would retreat to the basement. The next day, Mom's embarrassment was palpable as she had to borrow the neighbor's phone to schedule a repair.

Although my childhood fear was real, and the house was heavy with tension whenever Dad drank, he usually kept his temper from turning physical. Still, some painful incidents linger, and I would wager there were times he had no recollection of his behavior the next day.

When I was twelve, I was jolted awake one January night by a pounding on the kitchen door. Running downstairs, I saw Mom trying to get inside. It was three in the morning. The gold chain was latched across the door, preventing her from opening it. I quickly released the chain, and as she entered the room, she immediately stooped down to lie on the hard linoleum, writhing in pain. She was wearing thin nylon stockings, black high heels, and a short winter coat, and she was cold to the touch.

Frantic, I ran to get a cover. I laid down next to her, folding the blanket tightly around her. We were both crying. The story came out in bits and pieces.

"Pull the car over, Ray," she had said. "You've had too much to drink; let me drive." He stopped the car, but when she got out to walk around to the driver's side, he drove off.

Mom walked four miles home in the dark, cold winter night, alone and crying. The stores and bars were closed, and the streets were empty. She passed by pay phone booths, but without any money—not even a dime—she was unable to make a call.

As the story spilled forth, I realized Dad was sound asleep in their bed. He must have driven home, locked the door, and gone to bed. Later, Mom advised me that whenever I went out, I should carry money with me for emergencies. For me, though, the lesson embodied much more.

These memories spilled forth as I returned home after a two-year absence; it felt as if I had never left. I did not know how to name this feeling, but today, I might call it a kind of post-traumatic stress. Suddenly, I was overcome by a strong urge to escape, my body tense as feelings of helplessness and despair engulfed me.

Dan had just graduated from high school and was living at home, preparing to attend the Brown Institute in Minneapolis, where he anticipated a career in broadcasting, thanks to his deep, commanding voice. Lori was in high school, and Sissy, my sweet little sister with blonde ringlets and bright blue eyes, was only eight years old.

I wanted my mom to be happy, but I was at a loss on how to ease her burdens. "Mom, come out with Molly and me tonight. Molly said there is a good band playing at Diamond Jim's Supper Club."

"No, Kathi, I can't leave Sissy here alone with Lori; Dad might come home drunk."

"Mom, call your girlfriends and go out. I'll stay here and babysit Sissy," I begged. She refused my invitation. I was worried about her emotional state, pleading with her to talk to someone who might be able to help her.

Meanwhile, Mom turned her focus to me. I told her that two friends I had met while traveling in Europe were driving through Minnesota on their way to California and had invited me to join them. She encouraged me to go, even hosting them in our home before sending us off with plenty of food and sodas.

"Go, live your life, Kathi! I will be here when you return next year for nursing school."

So, I left. I spent the fall and winter in Wyoming and the summer in California. For my birthday greeting the next spring, Mom wrote:

Kath
Happy Birthday
My Heart is filled with love for you.
And filled with Great Big Wishes too.
For a Wonderful Year with Skies of blue and Sunshine Gleaming over you.
When evening falls with a Big Moon on high
May you look up with Stars in your eyes.
The Best is yet to come, my dear, yes, I predict a Most Wonderful Year!
You paid your dues
Forget the Blues, you deserve the best out there in the West.

*****

Returning to Minnesota in late summer of 1977 for nursing school, I was bursting with stories about my year out west. To my surprise, my perspective on Dad had softened; instead of anger, I felt sadness. Though he was still drinking, both my parents seemed more mellow, perhaps a result of Mom's quiet acceptance—or possibly, by her secret planning for a divorce. Living in Rochester, a short drive from St. Paul, allowed me to visit more frequently, during which I observed a fragile peace settle over their lives for the following two years.

In the fall of 1979, a few months after I began work as a registered nurse at the University of Minnesota Masonic Cancer Research Center, Mom's lawyer served Dad with divorce papers.

I was surprised by how upset Dad was when Mom initiated a divorce. He called me, wanting to set up a meeting. "It's urgent," he said. We met the next day in a small park along the Mississippi River Boulevard, where the leaves had already fallen off the trees, giving us a clear view of the murky river. The chill of the fall air met the coolness of my attitude toward Dad. I had thirty minutes before I had to be at the hospital for my afternoon shift.

After a quick hug, he started, "Kath—you know Mom has hired an attorney and filed for divorce." He paused, but stayed silent; it wasn't a question. "Mom listens to you. You've always been close. Would you please talk to her? Get her to change her mind. I love your mother; I don't want a divorce." He sounded on the verge of tears, but his eyes were dry.

The nerve, I thought. He actually asked me to talk Mom out of a divorce. I took a deep breath. "Dad," I started, "nothing I say will change Mom's mind. She has lived her life for you and her children. You've put her through a lot of pain. She is finally doing something for herself. I am proud of her and will support her decision." I tried not to scream; my heart was pounding.

Dad's facial expression turned to anger, then shifted back to sadness, but he remained silent. He knew I would not budge. After a few minutes, I said I had to get to work; I turned and walked to my car. I didn't look back. *Is Mom really going to do this?* I wondered.

A few days later, Dad had an appointment with his doctor, who confirmed a diagnosis of alcoholism and an enlarged liver. The physician advised him that if he continued drinking, he would likely die from cirrhosis. That awakening, coupled with Mom seeking a divorce, prompted him, once again, to promise Mom that he would quit drinking.

Every New Year's Day after a party night, Dad vowed to quit drinking. Sometimes, it lasted a week or two. Once, he was sober for five weeks. I lost hope in these empty promises. This time, though, he started attending Alcoholics Anonymous meetings. I stayed skeptical. But Mom stopped her divorce proceedings.

While he had fought his demons with alcohol for many years, Dad elected abstinence when he was forty-five years old. Thoughtfully, and with great effort, he tried to make up for lost time with his family, while maintaining a life of unvarnished sobriety.

It took some time, but I forgave Dad for the pain of my childhood; but forgiveness was harder for Mom. Her emotional scars ran deep. I know Dad's drinking affected my siblings, but I rarely discussed it with them. We each coped privately, much as we had been taught to do.

Mom reminded us that it was not appropriate to talk about family problems outside the home. I did, however, confide in Sister Diane when I was in sixth and seventh grades at St. Leo's elementary school. As a caring nun and teacher, she helped me navigate my confused feelings and anger. Now, I believe Mom would appreciate how telling my story, and hers, might be helpful to others.

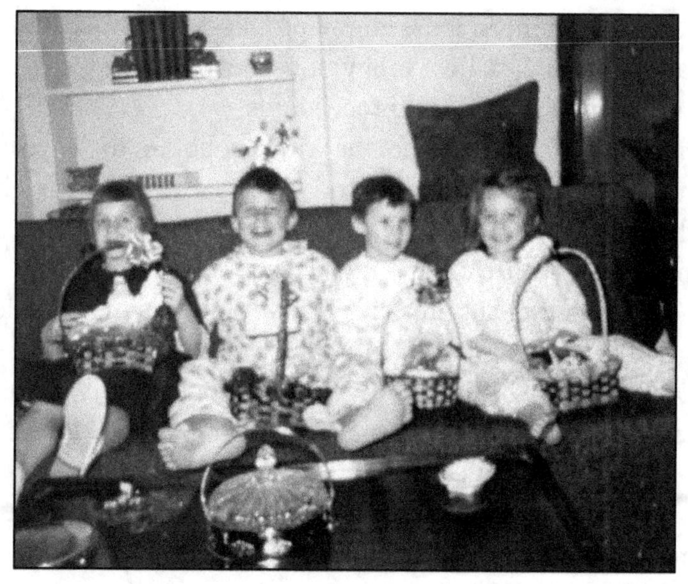

Cheri, Steve, Dan, and Kathleen sharing Easter fun

PART III

Signs of Diminishing Memory

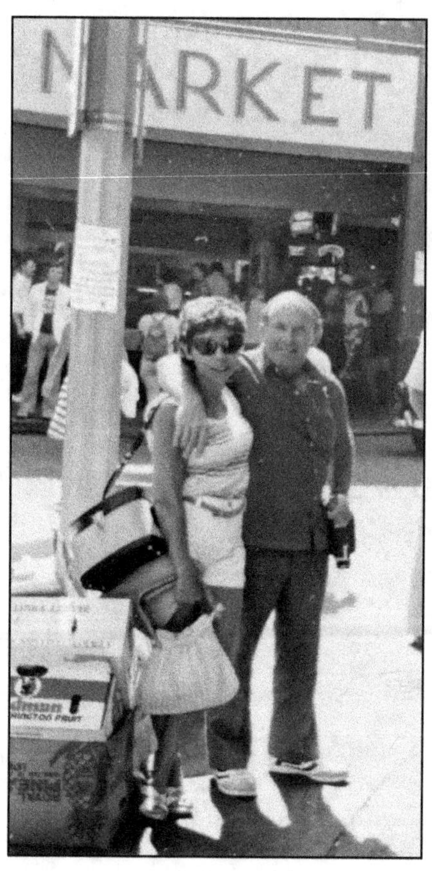

Mom and Dad at Pike Place Market in Seattle, 1982

5

Redefining Life

Mom took charge of her future after having raised her first five children. Taking care of people was her calling, so she became a home health aide. In March 1980, Mom was granted a diploma for completing the *Homemaker-Home Health Aide* program at the Saint Paul Area Technical Vocational Institute.

Enjoying her newfound independence, Mom searched personal ads in the local newspaper, the *Highland Villager,* seeking positions as a home caregiver. She was hired by many residents in the Highland Park area, where I grew up, which allowed her to stay close to home.

Mom's expertise was working with people who were homebound and needed assistance with their activities of daily living—also known as ADLs in the healthcare profession—such as bathing, dressing, feeding, and toileting. She also assisted with household chores while providing moral support and a sympathetic ear to family caregivers. Her clients often included elderly people living with dementia. As she shared some of their stories with me over the years, her love for her clients shone through her tears.

It was wonderful to see Mom's spirit shine and her self-confidence rise once she started working outside the home. The same year she received her diploma and her business began to flourish, my sister Lori married John, whom she had met at the Texaco station when he was working for Dad while attending carpentry school. John soon became like a third son to Mom and Dad. At twelve years old, Sissy was still at home. Since Dad was now sober, Mom felt comfortable leaving her with him in the evenings when she went out with a girlfriend.

During the first two years of Dad's sobriety, my witty boyfriend Ed and I spent many Saturday evenings playing cards with Dad. Mom, Sissy, Lori, and John joined in as well. Sometimes, rather than playing, Mom just enjoyed fussing over us, serving soda and snacks while listening to Ed's endless cache of jokes.

Meanwhile, I continued to work at the Masonic Cancer Center, where I nursed patients with leukemia and other metastatic cancers. I developed close relationships with many of my patients and their families, since in those days, patients essentially lived in the hospital for months while receiving a series of intensive chemotherapy treatments. Although the work was rewarding, the emotional toll was immense. I started dreaming about my patients, sometimes on the night they died, even while I was away on vacation. After two intense years of working in oncology, I was ready for a change.

During this period, I was communicating with a close friend in Seattle, who encouraged me to relocate there. With new opportunities in mind, I left Minnesota again, feeling confident that Dad's commitment to sobriety would endure, and Mom's work would continue to provide her with a sense of independence and happiness.

Once settled in Seattle, I embraced outdoor adventures, relishing the fresh, salty air and the enchanting scenery of snow-capped mountains and abundant waterways. I found nursing jobs were plentiful. The years flew by with annual visits back to Minnesota—and to my delight, one special vacation when my parents and two of my sisters came to visit and explore the Pacific Northwest with me.

*****

Seven years into Dad's sobriety, in the summer before Sissy entered college—solidifying Mom and Dad's status as empty nesters—Dad received shocking news. He was diagnosed with gall bladder cancer, which had spread into his liver.

The doctors informed him he had about six months to live. He accepted a trial of experimental chemotherapy, but the horrific side effects were unacceptable to him. He chose to live the time he had left without treatment, enjoying life as much as possible.

Mom took good care of Dad, just as she had cared for his dying mother, my grandmother Edith. I still marvel at how, when I was twelve years old, Mom nursed Edith for several months in our living room until her death. Before that, Edith had spent countless hours in bars, so we rarely saw her. Sometimes, she said mean things, so I kept my distance.

Years earlier, when Dad dated Mom, he introduced her to his mother by stopping in front of a bar. He told Mom he would be out in a minute. He came out with Edith, just as Mom was getting out of the car. She had barely said hello before Edith slid quickly back through the door into the dark bar. Dad told Mom then that he would not let alcohol control his life as his mother had—a hollow promise.

At the time of Dad's diagnosis, I was working as a registered nurse case manager in Seattle. For nearly every month of his illness, my flexible schedule allowed me to fly back to St. Paul for long weekends. During these visits, Dad confided in me that he believed God was punishing him with an early death. He expressed his great regret for not being a better Dad to me and a better husband to Mom. In those final months, we would sit together and talk.

Knowing I was coming home for Labor Day weekend, just weeks after Dad's diagnosis, Mom and Lori organized a family barbecue at Lori's house with all my siblings, their spouses, and my nieces and nephews. This gathering turned out to be one of the last times we were together as a family before Dad's health declined further.

In preparation for that visit, I flew home bearing gifts of flash-frozen salmon and halibut cheeks that my friend Jon had given me from his fishing work in Alaska. I hoped to rekindle good memories for Dad of their vacation to Seattle four years earlier, when he had eaten the delicious fish cooked many different ways. That trip was the first time I had had a vacation with my parents while Dad was sober.

Weeks later, in St. Paul again for a three-day Halloween celebration, I shared fun times with Mom and Dad. We dressed up in costumes and joined Lori's family for dinner. We also surprised Mom's oldest sister, my Aunt Gussie, with a visit. We wore brown paper bags over our heads that we had colored with scary, spooky faces. We knocked on Gussie's door and waited. Because it was nearly nine p.m. when we arrived, she cautiously peered through the locked porch screen door. Not recognizing us, but knowing we were not young children, she started reprimanding us for being out so late. We pulled the bags off our heads and yelled, "Trick or Treat!" Startled, it took her a minute to realize who we were. We had a good laugh followed by a lively visit.

The week before I traveled home for the Thanksgiving holiday, I called to inform Mom what time my plane would be arriving. "Oh, Kathi, are you coming home for the holiday weekend? I don't remember you telling me. You were just here for Halloween. How wonderful though! I'm so happy that we get to see you again so soon! What time should I pick you up?"

My mind filtered back to the past few conversations with Mom. I thought I told her I was coming home again. *Or did I just tell Dad?* She had me wondering. *Did I tell her? Did she forget I told her?* It was hard to imagine she would forget about my visit.

That Thanksgiving weekend, Dad asked me to take him to Saint Stanislaus Catholic Church, the same church he had attended as a youth. Although he didn't go regularly, he still held a strong affinity for the Catholic beliefs. When Dad committed to sobriety, he returned to Saint Stanislaus on a semi-regular basis and often met with Father Clay, who had helped him along his road to recovery. Located near downtown St. Paul, one block off West Seventh Street, the church was a sanctuary for him.

Specifically, Dad wanted me to accompany him to receive the Last Rites—a final anointing—from Father Clay. Knowing what this meant was heartbreaking; my eyes filled with tears. While I was honored that he invited me, it was painful that he didn't ask Mom. On the other hand, while Mom had a strong faith in God, she didn't share the deep-seated traditions that Dad revered—even though she had agreed to send their children to Catholic elementary schools.

On the drive home from the church, it became clear that Dad wanted time alone with me to discuss his concern about Mom. "I'm worried about your mom," he started. "She makes a grocery list, then leaves the house without it. She goes out to do several errands, but forgets to pick up my medication." He paused, looking at me with sadness in his eyes. "Once, she said she was going to start dinner, then an hour later, she asked me if she should order a pizza for us. I really think she is having trouble with her memory," he confided. "Have you noticed anything?"

While I did not share Dad's concern about these incidents because they seemed like absent-minded mistakes of a stressed caregiver and grieving wife, I did recall being surprised when Mom forgot that I was coming home this month. I shared this one episode, but said I hadn't noticed any other memory lapses. I acknowledged his concerns and promised to keep a close eye on her, sharing that I thought these episodes were the result of stress and grief. My impression was that his worry for Mom was heightened because he knew he would not be around to keep her safe.

Dad's appreciation for Mom was evident in the loving way he spoke about her. He looked at her with warmth and pulled her close, hugging her as if he didn't want to let go. He set out a hot cup of black coffee for her in the morning, while he made bacon and eggs. The sustained love between them was evident in the way she smiled and joked with him, as well as in the way they touched each other in passing.

Dad's death on January 14, 1987, left a void for his family and friends. He was just fifty-three. Mom was only fifty-two. I believed she had a whole new life waiting for her once she moved through her grief. I stayed with her for a couple of days after the funeral. I wondered about the paths Mom would forge and what dreams she might pursue next. I felt hopeful for her future.

Kathleen A. Hessler

6

Early Signs

After I returned to work in Seattle, I thought about Mom often, as she was living alone for the first time in her life with sole responsibility for finances and home. During our telephone conversations the month following Dad's death, I sensed she was overwhelmed navigating her life and working through her grief. Because of my concern, I returned home to Minnesota in late February for a ten-day visit.

While at home, I was helping Mom put groceries away in the kitchen cupboard. When she handed me a box of cereal, she asked, "Are you going to visit Cheri while you're home?"

"Yes, I plan to call her today," I said. "Will you come with me, Mom? I asked.

"Oh, no. I'm not up for a long drive in this winter weather," she responded.

"Okay, but the forecast looks mild. Please think about it. It would be fun to get away and spend some relaxing time together. We could even get a hotel for a night," I prompted, but she said nothing.

Then, she filled me in on recent news. There was much to catch up on in our large family. My siblings, all living in Minnesota, visited Mom frequently, and she often delighted in babysitting her growing number of grandchildren.

Her grief was visible when she spoke of my dad. She told me she missed him and that she had become accustomed to his presence. I could tell she was trying to be strong, despite the tears spilling down her cheeks. She said she had learned to relax and enjoy Dad's company again during his years of sobriety. I sensed she was grappling with the acceptance of his death and the void his absence created—especially after the renewed bond they had built. She shared that while she had sometimes confronted him about past harms, her love for him grew more and more as he demonstrated his remorse for the pain he had caused.

Mom asked again, "Are you going to see Cheri while you're here?" My older sister lived in a small town nearly three hours' drive north of St. Paul with her husband and children, so I didn't always have the opportunity to see her family when I visited.

"I hope so. I plan to call her today. Would you come with me, Mom?" I asked again, not wanting to point out that we had just discussed this.

"No, I'm not up for a drive," she said. We continued putting the groceries away in silence.

"Are you going to visit Cheri this week?" Mom asked again, ten minutes later.

"Mom, you've asked me that question three times in the last twenty minutes!" I snapped, surprised by my irritability.

She paused, looking confused. "Did I? I'm sorry, I think I have too much on my mind."

Later that day, as I reflected on our conversation, I was quick to attribute Mom's forgetfulness to the stress and grief of living on her own after thirty-four years of marriage. Certainly, settling into a life without Dad was causing her to be less attentive. I didn't dwell on it.

Nevertheless, that week, I discussed this incident with Lori. She revealed that shortly before Dad's death, he had expressed concerns about Mom's memory, just as he had to me. At that time, we both dismissed his fears, believing her memory lapses were due to the stress of caring for Dad.

Back in Seattle, I kept in close contact with Mom through heartfelt letters and phone calls, as we each worked through our grief.

*****

Over a year after Dad's death, Mom appeared to be healing and looking forward to new opportunities in life. She seemed happy while reconnecting with old friends in West Saint Paul, where she had gone to school with many Mexican Americans. She referred to Juanita as one of her "best chums." When Mom reconnected with her high school girlfriends, Juanita reintroduced her to her brother, Rodney. Mom shared that she had had a "crush" on him when she was young.

Mom and her friends enjoyed live music and dancing in the evenings. Rodney soon began spending time with the group, and Mom often talked about him and their mutual love of dancing. One week, she shared that they went out to dinner and a movie together— just the two of them. Her voice carried a lightheartedness I hadn't heard in years.

Through regular phone calls, I learned that Mom and Rodney spent many evenings out at dance clubs, igniting her passion for dance. When I asked about her time with him, she sounded young and carefree, eagerly reciting the recent movies they had seen and the bands they had heard. "We share the same love of movies and music," she'd say. "We both love jazz!" Her excitement was intriguing, as I couldn't recall the last time she had sparkled with such enthusiasm. Rodney took Mom to New Orleans a few times for long weekends where they danced well into the night. They also traveled to Las Vegas together; Mom, a self-professed "night owl," thrived in the nightlife.

As I listened to her stories, it became clear that dancing brought new meaning to her life. It was more than an activity for her; it was a way of helping her transform her grief into a renewed sense of purpose. I was happy for Mom.

Mom and Rodney frequented the Manor, a club located a couple of miles from her house. Several times during visits home, I would accompany them, smiling as I watched them whirl and spin on the dance floor. Mom, always impeccable in a fancy, colorful dress and high heels, looked dignified as she gracefully floated across the floor to a slow waltz.

"I love to dance," she whispered to me when she returned to the table. Rodney had whisked her off the dance floor when the band took a break. "Dancing is my favorite thing to do! I would give up everything just to be able to dance every night." Her smile was wide, and the light in her eyes shone brightly.

This was the first time in many years that I recalled seeing such passion and happiness in Mom's demeanor. Her joy was infectious. Even though I was hardly a seasoned dancer, I looked around the room for a lone gentleman who might want to dance. Seeing Mom this happy filled me with hope and helped me lift the past burdens of sadness I had carried for her. More than anything, I wanted her happiness to last.

7

Disorientation in Mexico: 1990

The hotel clerk summoned me to take a call from Mom. "We forgot my suitcase at the airport. What should we do?" Mom's anxious voice came through the receiver.

I had invited Mom and Rodney to join me in Mexico City for a few days before our planned trip to Puerto Vallarta. I had just completed six intense weeks studying international and immigration law during a summer program, and was looking forward to a much-needed break.

I was thrilled that Mom felt comfortable with the idea of traveling to Mexico with Rodney and for the opportunity to visit me there. Rodney's family was from Chihuahua, in northwestern Mexico, and his ability to speak Spanish helped ease her fear of being in a foreign country for the first time.

Mom always said she wanted to travel, but she believed she couldn't count on Dad to take care of us in her absence. I later realized she was afraid to venture anywhere new alone. Once, when I was trying to encourage her to get on a plane and travel by herself to my cousin's wedding in Wichita, she lashed out at me.

"Kathi, I'm not like you." Mom's voice rose as she emphasized her message. "I'm not comfortable traveling alone or being by myself in new places."

That statement surprised me. I had not realized Mom was uncomfortable traveling alone. She liked to explore and try new things, but I guess she wanted company. I reflected on this and realized how in tune she was with her children. She encouraged us to try new things, not wanting her fears to hold us back. So, I was happy when she had opportunities to travel with others.

In 1982, a year after Dad committed to sobriety, he and Mom visited me in Seattle with my sisters, Cheri and Sissy. During their week-long stay, we visited Pike Place Market and took a ferry to Bainbridge Island for a clam bake and Native American ceremony.

I reserved rooms in the well-known Edgewater Hotel on Elliot Bay, where, in 1964, the Beatles' visit put the hotel in the spotlight, marking its place in history. At the time of my family's visit, before liability lawsuits were rampant, one could still rent fishing equipment from the hotel, and guests could literally fish from their hotel window. I made sure Mom and Dad's room faced the water and that there was a fishing rod and bait in the room for Dad. My heart warmed when Mom's eyes brightened and her smile widened as she delighted in the beautiful view of the Puget Sound from their room.

Now, eight years after her trip to Seattle, I was thrilled to have Mom join me in Mexico. Mom and Rodney first landed in Mexico City, where I was completing my final exams. The plan was for us to spend two days sightseeing.

I had just completed one test and was back at my hotel getting ready to leave for my next exam when the hotel manager called. After Mom revealed that they were at the hotel, but her suitcase was at the airport, I was momentarily silent, trying to decide how to answer her question. *How do you forget a suitcase at the airport?* I wondered.

She had asked, 'What should we do?'

"Mom, Rodney speaks Spanish. Tell him to call the airport to ask if they'll deliver your luggage to the hotel. Or take a taxi back there to pick it up."

I did not understand why Rodney had Mom call me. This was something he should have been able to handle. Later, I reflected on this as I noticed his timid behavior about other things. In particular, I had asked Rodney to help me bargain in the open market for a purse, but he said he was not comfortable negotiating with the vendors, even though this was the custom, and he spoke Spanish.

Also, I realized I didn't know Rodney well. I think I had a false sense of comfort with him, knowing that Mom was enjoying life again and that his sister had been her high school friend. But what did I really know about him? Whenever I asked about his life, his answers were short. Perhaps this trip, we would have time to get to know each other better.

Later that day, after their suitcases were secure at the hotel and we sat down to eat dinner, toasting their trip with grand margaritas, I learned that Mom had forgotten her traveler's checks and credit card at home. I was stunned, unable to understand such forgetfulness. Yet, I was quick to rationalize it because Mom had been anxious about the trip, having never been out of the United States. Now, I had to figure out how to assist her with the money she would need on the trip. Back then, people going abroad would get traveler's checks at their banks because they were insured against loss.

One night the next week, after we had flown to Puerto Vallarta, Rodney and I were waiting in the patio bar of our hotel for Mom to come down for dinner. We were sipping margaritas, breathing in the fresh scent of colorful flowers, and basking in the warm ambiance of the decor. Mariachi singers were breaking out into song as they stopped at tables to serenade the guests. I glanced at my watch, not realizing how much time had passed. Mom tended to run late, so neither Rodney nor I had been concerned. I was enjoying the spirit of being on "Mexican time" after six weeks of study, but now worry clouded my thoughts.

Mom was always self-conscious about her appearance and made great efforts, like an artist, to apply her makeup and dress fashionably, often taking longer than planned. I usually allowed her extra time, but after over an hour of waiting, I suggested Rodney go check on her.

When they arrived at our table together fifteen minutes later, Rodney said that he found Mom wandering down the far end of the hall on the third floor of the hotel. Their room was on the fourth floor. Rodney said he mistakenly exited the elevator on the wrong floor and was about to reboard when he saw Mom cautiously walking down the hall toward him, confused. Mom brushed the whole event off, asserting the hotel had a confusing layout.

"Even Rodney got lost," she said, defending herself. "He got off the elevator on the wrong floor, too."

And it was a good thing he did, I thought.

We didn't speak of the incident again. I thought her explanation was plausible and didn't focus on it. This made sense to me; many hotels have confusing layouts, and it often takes a day or two to adjust to new surroundings. Later, Rodney told me in private that Mom admitted to him that she was lost, and just before he spotted her, he said she was starting to panic.

For the rest of our time in Puerto Vallarta, I kept a close watch on Mom. I noticed that she was frequently confused about her whereabouts. I thought back to the few days we were in Mexico City and her disorientation there. In the city, I was constantly guiding her in the right direction or pulling her back from walking across streets into oncoming traffic.

However, that was an easy one to explain away. Mexico City is a sprawling metropolis of over twenty million people who move around the massive city at all hours of the day and night. The noise, the traffic, the mixed smells of street food and exhaust—along with the foreign language—are enough to disorient many travelers.

In the following years, I would reflect back on this time as a foreshadowing of what was to come.

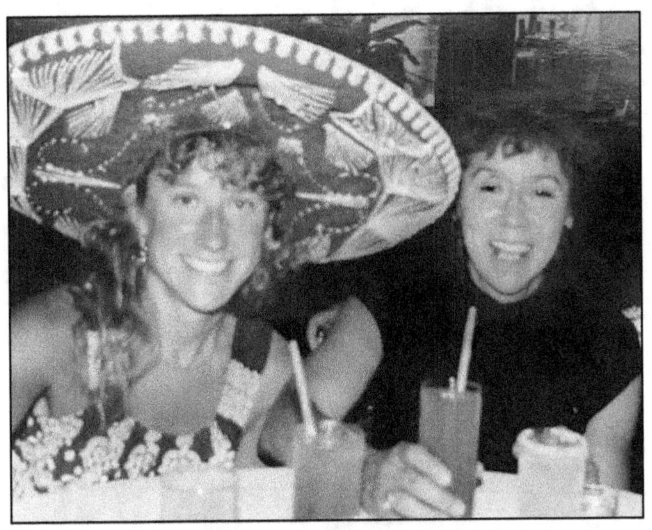

Kathleen and Mom in Mexico, 1990

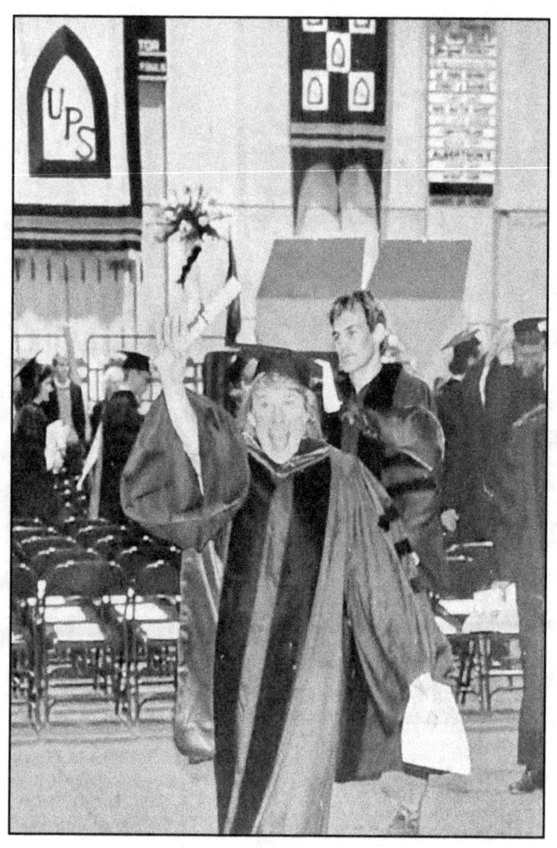

May 1991: Kathleen at Law School Graduation
Photograph by Leslie Gilpen Bateman

8

Law School Graduation: More Signs

May 19, 1991. My dream had finally come true. Mom and Rodney were there, cheering alongside my invited guests. My dear friend Leslie was in the back, snapping photos as I walked across the stage to receive my diploma at the University of Puget Sound School of Law in Tacoma, Washington.

Law school had been a long-held goal that took root in my teenage years at an all-girls, college-prep Catholic high school. We were told that women could further their education beyond high school and an undergraduate degree. It was in those classrooms that my aspirations for law school took hold.

While becoming a lawyer was my ambition, as life passed, my dreams were set aside to make room for other paths. Because I loved to travel, I studied nursing, which allowed me to work anywhere. Yet, deep inside, a strong drive pulled me toward law—the desire to advocate for justice. During Dad's sobriety, I shared my desire to become a lawyer, and he encouraged me to think more seriously about pursuing my dream. A little over a year after his death, in the summer of 1988, I entered the law program.

During law school, I worked full-time as a registered nurse in Seattle and commuted nearly an hour south to Tacoma four nights a week for classes throughout the year. Carpooling with three other students made the drive pass quickly as we discussed cases and quizzed each other. Weekends were devoted to studying after brisk morning runs and breakfast with friends. After three years, I walked with the other graduates, feeling a great sense of relief.

My friends, many of them physicians, nurses, nutritionists, and pharmacists, were there to celebrate. Several of the women, who were my running buddies, completed a marathon that morning in nearby Olympia, Washington. When they finished the race, the group headed to my graduation ceremony to watch my rite of passage that would take me from nursing to opportunities in the legal community.

After the graduation ceremony, the warm, sunny day allowed everyone to gather outside for visiting and picture taking—freeze-framing moments one click at a time. When I look back at those photographs and recall the images imprinted in my memory, I see Mom standing alone off to the side, though she was near my group of friends. Her eyes were blank; she seemed lost and disoriented, staring into the crowd. I had introduced her to my friends and moved around to speak with others.

When I turned to look back, I was struck by Mom's unusual demeanor and look of bewilderment. The exuberant crowd noise faded for a moment. My earlier happiness was marked with sudden concern. Not wanting to dwell on this troubling moment, I turned back to the crowd of students huddled with family and friends, absorbing the shouts of "Congratulations! I knew you could do it! Way to Go!" The blue sky shined bright, a gift to graduates who had spent many gray, rainy days in the library—but for me, it had lost some of its shine.

Mom could be shy in a crowd; self-conscious was really the word for it. Still, it was odd for her not to engage with others. While her self-esteem had suffered from years of living with an alcoholic, she had always been comfortable making conversation with my friends. As I watched her from a distance, I saw my boyfriend, Axel, approach her. I did not see Rodney anywhere.

Axel lived in Seattle's Ballard neighborhood. His mother, who had lived next door to me for many years, introduced us when I was in law school. His parents had immigrated to America from northern Germany when Axel was three years old. His father, a master sailmaker, started a sailmaking business, which Axel and his brother Frank inherited.

The day Mom and Rodney arrived, I took them to Schattauer Sails so Mom could meet Axel and get a tour of the loft, which boasted many stories. The display of handwritten postcards told the tales of their customers who had thrived in various exotic places after sailing away from Seattle with their new custom cruiser sails. I could tell that Mom and Rodney enjoyed learning about Axel's trade by the way they talked about the visit several times that weekend.

Now, Axel, always a gentleman, took my mom by the arm and led her to me as I said goodbye to friends, reminding them where to go for the dinner celebration in Seattle.

An hour later, we were at Louie's Cuisine of China, a neighborhood restaurant just north of the Ballard Bridge. I reserved a room for twenty-five people. The tables were arranged in a large U-shape, allowing everyone to see each other. Mom sat on my left side with Axel on my right.

During the festivities, while I chatted with Axel, I was conscious of Mom. Although Rodney sat to her left, she wasn't conversing with him. I leaned forward, looking inquiringly into Rodney's eyes, hoping for some interaction. He shook his head. I nodded as Mom gazed at the room, silent, staring. Brushing aside my feeling of her hollowness, I spoke to her. She answered with short responses, almost mechanically.

I experienced an eerie sense that she was not truly present. It is difficult to describe: the memory of that dinner sticks with me like a heavy meal, the sense of her emptiness pressing on my heart. The feeling lodged itself in my chest. Yet, even as these emotions arose, I did not understand what was wrong and did not express my concern to her.

The entire trip, however, was not discouraging. Mom rallied and engaged in other conversations and activities. She readily expressed her opinions when we were alone or with a smaller group.

We shared a lively adventure at Seattle's Pike Place Market, where she was engaged and interested in the bustling scene. She talked of her visit with Dad and my sisters eight years earlier. We were captivated by the show put on by the famous fish vendors, who tossed large, silvery salmon into the air from one fishmonger to another, shouting out the prices while trying to promote sales. I marveled at the heaps of fresh shrimp and clams, the mussels and Dungeness crab, and the large, meaty Alaskan King Crab legs—all resting on mounds of crushed ice.

The fish smells lingered until we reached the sweet aromas of the flower and food vendors. We walked at a leisurely pace alongside the merchants' booths, enjoying the vibrant colors of the fruits and vegetables—robust red tomatoes, large green apples, clusters of plump, purple grapes, and bundles of blackberries.

We dawdled at the craft booths, admiring the carved wooden products, including Native American totems, creative one-of-a-kind jewelry designs, and unique articles of clothing. There were souvenirs of the rainy city, including umbrellas and T-shirts marked with famous Seattle emblems. At the end of the row of vendors, we stopped to enjoy the breathtaking view of Elliot Bay and the ferryboat crossing the Puget Sound westward, toward Bainbridge Island.

Mom loved to shop, so after we left Pike Place Market, we stopped at well-known downtown Seattle stores. Nordstrom's was a must. At times, Mom's face betrayed her moments of confusion, but I dismissed it, thinking she wasn't an experienced traveler. I reflected on our trip to Mexico the previous summer, but would not allow myself to dwell on any troubling thoughts. Rodney was easy-going, almost passive, and went along wherever we ventured.

Mom and Rodney stayed with me at the house I had rented for eight years, in the Phinney Ridge area of Seattle. My roommate at that time was Susan; she was friendly and kind to my mom and Rodney. The house was old and somewhat rundown, but it was quaint and had a fabulous western view of the Olympic Mountains from the large deck where I hosted many fun dinner parties. It was pleasant to sit outside in the mornings, looking out at the Seattle greenery and the snow-capped peaks to the west.

One morning, while Mom was in the shower and Rodney was taking a walk, Susan shared a story with me. She had asked my mom if she was enjoying her stay in Seattle, and Mom replied, "Yes, but I wish I could get a decent cup of coffee around here."

We laughed over that. Mom, having grown up with the coffee products of the 1950s and 1960s, loved her brewed Maxwell House or Folgers' coffee. Apparently, she was unaware that Seattle, with the birth of Starbucks in the 1970s, had become the coffee capital of the United States.

So, I went out and bought her a can of Maxwell House to brew at home. However, first, I took her to Starbucks and introduced her to lattes. Several years later, she would come to enjoy this special coffee drink with flavorful syrups that my sisters and I would bring to her.

When I met up with friends a few days after Mom's visit to Seattle, they were happy to see me, but also worried. While they said they enjoyed meeting my mom, they eventually shared their concern about her. They were forthcoming, each with a different question.

"Your mother didn't seem well to me. Does she have medical problems?"

Another friend asked, "Does your mother have problems with alcohol—is she a heavy drinker?"

A third friend inquired, "Is your mom experiencing side effects of medications she might be taking? Or, do you think she might have a drug addiction?"

The questions were varied, but alarming. My friends and I had observed the same demeanor, but they all had different thoughts as to what might be causing her behavior. As I listened to them, troubling thoughts grew in my mind: Was Mom struggling with a serious medical issue that I failed to notice? I needed to understand what was wrong.

Although it may have seemed insensitive, my friends inquired in a loving manner. Because so many of them, like me, were healthcare professionals, they were comfortable being direct with me about their observations. I knew the answers to their questions were a resounding "no," but I did not know what was wrong.

A few days later, I would be traveling back to Minnesota for Sissy's wedding, where I would be able to observe Mom in her own surroundings. I had put the date on my calendar many months ago, looking forward to celebrating my youngest sister's wedding. Now, my purpose in going home would be twofold.

As usual, when in St. Paul, I would stay with my mom. This allowed me time to visit with her alone and to assess how she was managing. Although I would only be able to stay for a long weekend, I planned to focus on her well-being.

9

What is Wrong?

The weekend in St. Paul was filled with pre-ceremony activities. We were grateful that it was sunny with temperatures in the low 70s, so that Sissy's special wedding day would shine bright in all our memories. Mom and I kept busy helping with last minute preparations, and I took her to her beauty shop appointment.

Reflecting on what I had witnessed in Seattle and the inquiries from my friends, I arrived in St. Paul on high alert to observe my mom and note any lapses in memory, withdrawal during social events, or episodes of confusion. I also wanted to speak with my sister Lori to hear if she had experienced any unusual incidents with our mother. The fear of what I might discover occupied my mind, casting a shadow over the weekend.

I spent as much time as I could with Mom, driving us to activities and to the wedding. Of course, Rodney went with us everywhere because he didn't have a driver's license. When I asked why Rodney didn't drive, my mom explained that he had been in an accident in his youth and never wanted to drive again. She asked me not to discuss it with him.

At the reception, I noticed Mom seemed confused about where we were sitting after using the ladies' room. It wasn't unusual since there were many people, perhaps over a hundred, who came to celebrate Sissy and Brian, and it was the first time she had been to the venue. For the most part, because we were in her familiar surroundings over the weekend, she seemed quite at ease.

On my last day in town, I had the opportunity to speak with Lori. I briefed her on my observations from the previous week in Seattle—Mom's confusion and occasional odd behavior—as well as what some of my friends had said. I asked Lori if she, or any of our other siblings, had noticed changes in Mom's memory during the past year. After Mom's trip to Mexico a year earlier, I had discussed her confusion and forgetfulness with Lori. However, I did not focus on it because I believed her confusion was the result of traveling in a foreign country for the first time.

This time, Lori immediately told me about a situation that occurred more than a year earlier. "Kath," she said, "did I ever tell you about when I asked Mom to babysit Andrea and Joe?" She didn't pause long enough for me to respond. "John and I were going to his brother's wedding in Houston, so a month in advance, I asked Mom to babysit for the three-day weekend. She'd agreed to come stay with the kids that weekend."

She paused before continuing. "Mom called me every day for over a week, remembering her commitment to babysit, but not the dates. I suggested she mark the dates on the calendar I had purchased and placed on the door in her kitchen."

"I remember you telling me about this," I said.

Lori continued, "On one of my visits to Mom's house, I looked at the calendar and saw that she still hadn't marked the weekend we were going to be gone, so I filled in the dates with a bold black marker. Prior to leaving town, I called Denise, my neighbor who lives across the street, and shared my concerns about Mom. She agreed to check on her and the kids several times a day and in the evenings. Thankfully, Denise was there each time I called that weekend. I also alerted my next-door neighbor, Heather, for added vigilance."

After that experience, Lori did not ask Mom to babysit the kids again for any length of time. It was hard to reconcile these types of events when much of her life seemed normal, and she was often engaged in fruitful conversation and activities.

Following her weekend away in Houston, Lori talked with our other siblings to see if anyone else had observed lapses in Mom's memory while spending time with her. Nothing notable was mentioned. As everyone navigated their busy lives, they monitored Mom when they spent time with her, updating Lori on any unusual incidents that occurred. Time had sped by with no major reports that year except for my graduation weekend.

Trying to separate these unusual occurrences, which seemed far apart in time and space, I ruminated on Mom's work life. She loved her clients, and for several years after Dad's death, she continued to respond to ads in the local neighborhood newspaper, juggling several people at a time. She visited each client two or three times a week and assisted them with their ADLs. Sometimes, they asked if she would shop for food or household items, and because they trusted her, they gave her their credit cards.

At the time of Sissy's wedding, Mom shared that she was only working with one client at a time—rather than two or three, which had been her norm. I saw that she had written the days of the week and the time she was scheduled to be at her client's home on her calendar. She must have realized her own limitations by decreasing her client load, but was unwilling to give up the work she loved completely.

Mom had always taken a genuine interest in people. Molly, a dear friend of mine since grade school, told me that my mom was "a friend to my friends." Molly said that whenever she called my house when we were young, or when I was home visiting as an adult, Mom would ask her questions about her life.

"Your mom was different from most moms," Molly said to me one day. "I could tell she was genuinely interested in me and in what was going on in my life. Other friends' parents weren't like that. It meant a lot to me."

As a compassionate caregiver, Mom often expressed her concern about how her clients and families would manage in the long term. Over the course of ten years working with elderly and infirm people, she gained firsthand experience caring for patients with memory loss. She became knowledgeable about the warning signs and symptoms of dementia. Based on her clients' struggles and her role supporting them, she understood the devastating impact a diagnosis of Alzheimer's has on both the patient and their family.

The months following my graduation and Sissy's wedding, Mom contemplated whether her increasing episodes of forgetfulness could be signs of Alzheimer's disease. She started to talk about it, calling me often. She would voice her fears; her trembling words, filled with desperation, pierced my heart.

"Kathi, what if I have this disease? What *will* I do? What *will* I do?" Her voice trailed off into stifled, muffled cries.

"Mom, what does your doctor say?" There was silence on the phone line. I knew the doctor hadn't offered much, but I wanted to hear if she remembered anything from her visits. I continued, "I know Lori went with you to see your doctor. I will call her to talk about what she learned. Maybe it isn't Alzheimer's. It could be something treatable. Recently, you told me you fell and hit your head hard on the ice last winter."

I didn't have any answers, especially since the most recent visit with Mom's family practice physician had yielded no recommended actions except to continue monitoring her symptoms. In the early 1990s, physicians were hesitant to diagnose Alzheimer's in patients who could still function in their daily lives. Back then, the diagnosis relied on a person's symptoms and eliminating other causes of memory loss because the only definitive way to confirm Alzheimer's was by performing a brain biopsy after death. While that remains true today, there are more sophisticated tests to determine a likely diagnosis of Alzheimer's. Still, ruling out other causes of memory loss is important. Such causes may include: medication side effects, vitamin deficiencies, thyroid disorders, or brain injuries.

*****

Returning to Seattle, I focused on studying for my Washington State law license. The test was offered twice a year. In late July, after the three-day grueling examination, I explored job options in healthcare law while continuing to work at Ballard Community Hospital. My goal was to secure an in-house attorney position with a large healthcare provider. I sent out resumes and scheduled informational interviews while networking at legal and healthcare events in the Seattle area.

Throughout the summer, I made a point to communicate with my siblings about Mom. By late August, we became more aware of Mom's progressive memory issues when we exchanged information as troubling incidents became more frequent.

In September 1991, Sissy and Lori took Mom, accompanied by Rodney, to see Dr. Susan Smith, a Clinical Neuropsychologist. Dr. Smith evaluated Mom and listened as my sisters provided a detailed medical and behavioral history. She concluded that Mom's symptoms were likely due to an organic process—an indication of physical or biochemical changes in the brain leading to cognitive impairment. She suspected possible Alzheimer's disease but emphasized that a certain diagnosis could not be made because there was no single test or biomarker for Alzheimer's. Dr. Smith noted Mom's recent fall, but explained that a previous CT scan had shown no unusual findings, a result described in the report as "unremarkable." Given the examination results, the neuropsychologist recommended that Mom only drive when accompanied by someone. Alternatively, she suggested that Mom not drive at all.

Although it was a blessing that Mom had voluntarily stopped seeing clients that summer, we were uncertain how to manage this situation, because Mom engaged appropriately much of the time and was aware of her surroundings.

10

Taking Away the Car

Despite our busy lives, my siblings and I talked often, sharing more of Mom's memory lapses. We needed a plan—especially after receiving the written report from Dr. Smith. The results were sobering, specifically her recommendation that Mom not drive. But Dr. Smith offered no guidance on how to proceed. *How should we approach this? Who will take the lead?*

Over the previous year, I had learned about Alzheimer's by reading books and consulting with healthcare professionals in my job. Meanwhile, my siblings gained knowledge through reading and attending classes. Yet, with no clear direction from Mom's care providers, we were struggling through a maze of information and uncertainty. Time marched on as we watched and wondered what to do, still without a definitive plan. Instead, we reacted with Band-Aids when Mom's behaviors sounded an alarm or raised a safety concern.

On one occasion, Lori invited Mom over to her house for dinner after she finished her weekly beauty shop appointment. Not only did Mom arrive late, but Lori noticed that her hair was a mess. "Mom, I thought you said you were going to the hair salon today?" Lori asked.

"I was…," Mom slowly admitted, then said, "Lori, I drove around for two hours, and I couldn't find the beauty shop!" Mom started to cry. The hair salon was a place she had frequented for fifteen years.

Lori asked more questions. Mom eventually admitted she had trouble finding Lori's house and was getting lost more often in familiar surroundings. My brother Dan then recounted an earlier event: Mom called him one day from a phone booth in a panic, saying she didn't know where she was. After talking to her for a few minutes,

Dan realized she was in Highland Park near the Powers department store. He picked her up and drove her home.

These incidents created a sense of urgency. We knew for certain that Mom was getting lost, and we were increasingly concerned about her driving and the safety of others. Despite understanding the seriousness of the situation, none of us wanted to be the "bad cop."

Recognizing the need to take Mom's car away, Lori and I discussed the possibility of asking Ken Rhodes, Dad's former business lawyer and estate planner, to help us. He and his wife had been Mom and Dad's friends. I knew Mom would listen to and respect what Ken had to say. I called and explained the situation. He expressed sympathy on hearing about Mom's condition. He said she had stopped by his office many months before to ask him some questions about her will, and he noticed then that she was having trouble finding the right words, and something felt off.

I asked if he would make an appointment with Mom at her home to talk to her again about business issues, then shift the conversation to her memory and the dangers of driving with memory loss. Thinking it would be more humiliating for my mom if I were at the house, I asked if he thought it best for him to go alone. He did.

Shortly before Ken's visit, I flew home from Seattle for a few days, but I was conveniently out doing errands when Ken arrived at Mom's house on that fateful day. Before I left, I reminded her that she had an appointment with Ken written on her calendar—that he would be visiting with her when I was out.

After Ken left that day, I returned from errands with a bag of groceries. Mom greeted me at the door, crying. "This is the worst day of my life!" Mom spoke loudly, dabbing at her tears with a tissue.

She screamed at me. "This is the worst day of my life! This is a horrible day! Where were you? Did you see Ken? He just left. He took my car keys and told me I shouldn't be driving anymore." She was shaking; her sobbing and anguish brought tears to my eyes.

"No, Mom, I didn't see him." He must've left a few minutes before I arrived. "Mom, tell me about your visit. What did Ken say?"

Mom shouted, "Ken came over to talk to me about driving. He said he was concerned about me because the last time we met, I was having trouble staying focused on our conversation. I confided in him about some of my recent problems. Then he said it would be safer for me not to drive anymore! I was so surprised and upset, but I felt I didn't have a choice when he asked for my car keys. This is the worst day of my life! The worst day of my life! He told me I shouldn't be driving anymore. Did you hear what I said?"

I was silent for several seconds. "Yes, Mom. I'm so sorry." Her devastation pierced my heart.

"What will I do without a car? What will I do?" The tears were streaming down her face, the mascara darkening the circles under her eyes. "How will I get around? I just lost my freedom!" She sobbed that day and would for many more.

Mom didn't learn to drive until I was ten years old; we could count on her being home after school. We were accustomed to walking the mile to and from school every day unless a neighbor offered us a ride.

Prior to getting her license, Mom did her shopping from the Sears and Montgomery Ward catalogs. She also called Clemens' grocery store on St. Clair to order our weekly food staples. Dad serviced all Clemens' trucks and plowed the store parking lot in the winter. Most weeks, he would pick up the order on his way home from work, but on several occasions, Mr. Clemens delivered the groceries to our home. Mom lamented the fact that she couldn't conduct her own errands, so she took a driver's education course.

On the day Mom passed her driver's test, while walking home from school, I saw a gray car turn the corner onto our street, Norbert Lane. The person honked at me, but I couldn't see who was in the car. A few minutes later, when I turned the corner and saw the dark gray Dodge Dart in our driveway, I hurried my pace, excited because I thought we had company. As I rushed into the house, Mom greeted me with a beaming smile and a big hug.

"Did you see me turn the corner a few minutes ago? I got my driver's license today! And Dad bought me a car. We're going out to eat at Burger King tonight. We'll get Whoppers and celebrate! Dad won't be home until late because he's bowling tonight."

Still recalling the joy on her face that day long ago, I sat with Mom after Ken had taken her car keys. We discussed ways she could continue to live independently without relying on driving.

"What'll Rodney and I do? He doesn't drive," she cried. I reminded her that Rodney is experienced with the St. Paul bus system. We talked about how they could still go dancing at the Manor, just a few miles away, by taking a bus or cab. The movie theater was within walking distance. I reminded her that Lori lived five miles away and she was able to take her on errands and to medical appointments.

After that day, Lori stopped by more frequently with her children, dropping off groceries and household supplies. These visits gave Andrea and Joey time with Grandma while Lori checked for safety hazards at the house.

*****

We were not alone in dealing with this issue. Many families struggle with taking keys away from family members with dementia. Years after we experienced this heart-wrenching decision with Mom, I was practicing law, representing the continuum of long-term care entities. In my practice, I saw that this was a common issue for seniors in independent living apartments.

I remember a particularly poignant incident. A client who operated a continuing care retirement community called me for advice. The community director described a resident who was experiencing progressive dementia. The woman lived in the independent living apartments. My client had arranged a meeting with the resident's adult children to communicate her concerns about their mother's well-being.

At the meeting, the director urged the children to take their mother's keys away, or at least hide them. She recommended several options: one of the children could ask to "borrow" the car for a few weeks, or they could call the Department of Motor Vehicles (DMV) to report her. Alternatively, they could contact their mother's physician and request that he report her to the DMV. The director warned, though, that there could be a delay before DMV acted. This discussion set the stage for the difficult decisions the family faced.

The resident was still living independently, so the retirement community could not legally intervene to take away her keys. They did the next best thing by convening the meeting. Additionally, the director suggested working together to help their mother transition into assisted living within the community.

The children were reluctant to confront their mother or work out a plan. They wanted to think about it.

Regrettably, two weeks later, with keys in hand, the woman left the community and drove the wrong way onto the freeway, causing a tragic accident that killed a young man. The resident also died. At that point, I was asked to investigate the matter to ensure my client had taken all necessary actions required under the law.

*****

It was painful and heartbreaking to see Mom's devastation at losing her freedom to drive. Still, it was important to think about her safety and the well-being of everyone on the road. My heart was heavy with sadness for her.

Mom remembered that day for a long time; she asked me from time to time if she had ever told me about "the worst day" of her life. It was a turning point. While my mom slowly adjusted to this traumatic life change, she still continued to grieve the loss of driving—which was a sign of her vanishing independence.

In the weeks after that awful day, my brother Dan helped with the sale of her car. He told me he would never forget the anguish on Mom's face when the new owner drove the car out of her driveway and down the road, out of sight forever.

11

Discussion about Advance Directives

Mom was fidgeting, getting up every few minutes, and asking if she could get me anything—even though we were sitting at the dining room table amidst an array of food and a pot of freshly brewed coffee. It was late summer 1992, and I had planned this visit to talk about advance directives.

"Mom, please sit down with me and enjoy a cup of this fresh coffee. It's the perfect temperature."

"Okay," she said and sat down with her cup. She put a cinnamon roll—one of her favorite sweets—on a small plate.

"Mom, I'm worried about you. I know you visited your doctor and a clinical specialist about your memory. But they haven't offered you any definitive advice on living with your memory loss or given you any treatment options. I want to help you. We love you; we all worry about you living alone." I hesitated.

"I know you do, but I'm managing okay. I don't want to think about it—my memory. I'm not driving anymore. Did I tell you about the day Ken came over and took my car keys?" There was a long pause. "It was the worst day of my life!"

"I know, Mom. I'm so sorry." We sat in silence.

Fortunately, she was lucid that day, so I took the opportunity to discuss future planning. One confusing aspect about Alzheimer's disease is that a person may have prolonged cogent periods where everything appears normal. People who interacted with Mom briefly, such as in a grocery store or restaurant, may not notice anything unusual about her behavior. She followed conversations and often responded appropriately.

Similarly, it was not unusual for Mom to converse long-distance by telephone for hours with her older brothers, Bill and Alex, and her sister-in-law, Gloria. For a long time, my aunts and uncles were unable to detect any abnormalities in their conversations with her. But they typically reminisced about the past when they spoke.

Often, in the early stages of the disease, long-term memory remains intact while short-term recollections deteriorate. Mom's course was following this pattern. It is during this time that many people with dementia often develop coping mechanisms—called social graces—to mask their forgetfulness. They might say things like, "Oh yes, that's exactly what I was going to say," or, "Yes, just what you said! Exactly."

When she was thinking clearly, Mom wanted to talk and plan. But she was frightened, and I wasn't sure she knew how to express her fear or ask for help. We sat in silence. I searched for the right words, but found none. Then she spoke with a quiver in her voice.

"I'm scared," she said, her eyes moistening. "I told you about Albert, the last man I cared for in his home. He was very confused, and I could tell that his memory was failing him. He would ask me for breakfast right after I finished cleaning him up from his morning meal. I'm afraid that might happen to me."

Her voice became calm as she talked more about Albert. "Kathi, you would have loved Albert. He was so sweet. It was so sad that he didn't know his wife, Martha. He called her Annie. Annie was their daughter who died in a car accident as a teenager. I helped Martha bathe Albert and stayed with him while she ran out to do errands. I can't imagine what it must've been like living with him—taking care of him twenty-four hours a day."

Mom stopped talking, and her eyes welled up. I waited. "What will I do if this happens to me? Who will help me?" She cried softly.

I got up and went to her, hugging her tightly. "Mom, let's talk about this. We can all help you. We want to help you. If you let me, or Lori, be your durable power of attorney, this would allow us to help you pay your bills and take care of any necessary business issues."

"You mean, give you access to my checkbook and bank accounts?" She stopped crying and looked up questioningly.

I answered, "Yes, but we'd only write a check or use your account if you want us to help you pay your bills. I know Lori visits you twice a week and brings you groceries. And if you need more help at home, we can have someone come in to help you."

"I don't want anyone to come into my house!" She started to get angry.

"Mom, I know you don't, but remember how much your clients and their families enjoyed your company and looked forward to having you come into their homes to help them. Your help allowed them to live at home instead of having to move." I almost said "into a nursing home," but stopped. I wasn't ready for this.

"Help me understand. I'm not sure I need this." She was calm and quite logical.

"Mom," I continued, "many people in good health have durable powers of attorney and a separate document naming an agent to make healthcare decisions for them if it becomes necessary. It's the smart thing to do—to plan ahead." I paused, and she looked at me intently, like she expected me to continue.

"For example, if you had a stroke and you were temporarily unable to pay your bills or make a decision about healthcare treatment, even for a short time, the person you choose as your durable power of attorney and healthcare agent will take over for the period of time you are unable to make decisions for yourself. Once you are well, you make your own decisions again." I was trying to decide if she understood.

"I see," she said. "Your dad didn't have anything like that when he was sick." She made a good point. She was following the conversation.

"You are right, Mom. When people are married, it is often accepted that the spouse will make choices for the other in cases where one is unable to make their own decisions. Also, the law has changed since Dad died. It now allows you and me, or anyone of legal age, to fill out a document called a Power of Attorney for Healthcare and a Living Will form that tells the doctor what treatments or care you would want should you have a life-threatening illness." I paused.

"Like what?"

"Well, an example of a drastic situation would be if you had a car accident that resulted in a brain injury, and the only way you could continue to live is with a ventilator. Some people call it a respirator, because a ventilator is a machine that helps you breathe. The law allows a person to say, in advance, that if they were in such a situation, they would not want the doctors to keep them alive on a ventilator." I stopped talking.

"I see," Mom said in a contemplative voice.

"Mom, do you know that some people in comas, or others who are on ventilators, have a feeding tube inserted into their stomach to provide them with food and nutrition? The person is then fed with liquid food and water placed through the feeding tube."

She was quick to reply. "I would never want that!"

Her reply led to further discussion about what she would want if her appointed agent had to speak on her behalf. She stopped crying and was calm, apparently comprehending this information.

"Will you do this for me? Be the person who would make these decisions?" She looked at me with her deep brown eyes and waited.

"I would be happy to do this for you, Mom, but since I live in Seattle, it may be a good idea if I do it with Lori, especially since she lives so close to you and visits you often. We would then be co-agents for you. What do you think of that idea?"

"I suppose we should do this," she said, her voice trailing softly.

We needed to do this sooner, rather than later, while Mom still had the capacity to make these decisions. Her longer, lucid periods were decreasing, and I did not want to go to the courts for an appointment of a conservator or guardian.

The process of achieving a court-appointed conservatorship (for financial decisions) or guardianship (for decisions over the person, such as healthcare decision-making) can be expensive and detrimental to both the family and the patient, especially if the court appoints a stranger. The guardian stranger may act in a hostile manner toward the family and exclude them from important decisions. Going to court should be a last resort.

Because of these dangers, it is preferable that a person, when of sound mind, make the decision in advance about who they would want to serve as their durable power of attorney and agent for healthcare decision-making. It is almost always best if the appointed person or people are trusted individuals with close family ties.

In late summer of 1992, I spoke to Ken Rhodes again. I asked him to visit Mom and help her understand these documents and what she needs to do to satisfy Minnesota law.

Within weeks of our discussion, Ken met with Mom to execute these documents. Lori and I officially became Mom's co-agents for financial and healthcare decisions. We handled issues together as they arose, and through our concerted efforts, we were able to continue helping Mom so she could remain in her own home for now.

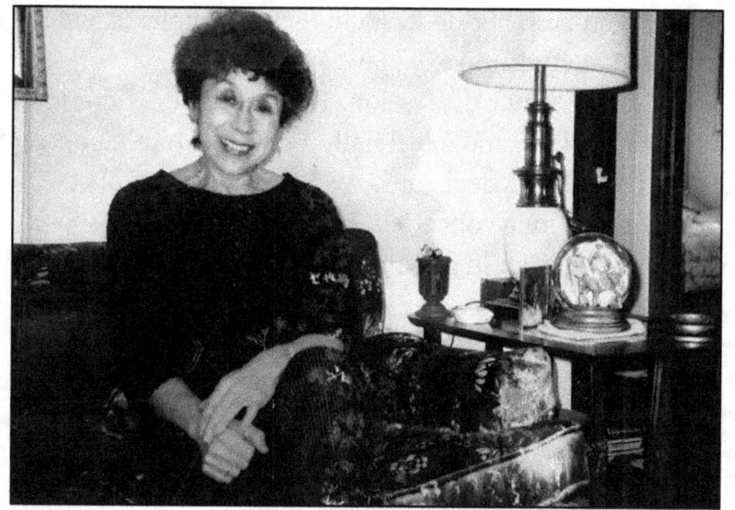

Mom's favorite couch

12

Delusions and Disarray

Each time I returned to visit Mom over the next two years, I noticed unusual clutter, such as piles of papers and unopened mail left on the table or counter. Sometimes, the furniture was dusty, and dishes and clothes lay scattered, revealing a pattern of disarray. This was so unlike her. She had always kept a clean and organized home, even though we had grown up in crowded quarters.

Mom lived in the same three-bedroom house we had moved to when I started second grade. The upstairs was one large room that I shared with my three sisters, while my two brothers shared a small one with bunk beds down the short hall from my parents' bedroom on the main floor. The lone bathroom was set between the two. When I was a teenager, Dad added a shower in the basement laundry room.

The kitchen, dining room, and living room were small. The dining table nearly filled the entire room; we had to be careful when pulling the chairs away from the table to avoid scraping the wall. Whenever I returned home, I pondered how we managed getting ready for work or school with only a single bathroom. Moreover, I was in awe at how Mom had managed to keep an immaculate home with the comings and goings of growing teenagers. As I thought about the emotional burdens she endured, I found it admirable.

Now, Mom's small rat terrier dog wandered the house freely. Previously, Penny knew her place was downstairs in the recreation room. On the main level, she was only allowed to sit by the kitchen door. If she wandered farther, she was inevitably reprimanded. But things had changed—Mom now ignored Penny's advances into the rest of the house—as the clever dog had become her dearest companion.

During one visit home, I was looking for the portable telephone to make a call. Mom didn't remember where she put it. She was moving about the main floor annoyed, searching everywhere. Frustrated that she had misplaced it, she became obsessed with finding the phone. I attempted to distract her.

"Mom, would you like some ice cream?" I yelled from the kitchen into the bedroom, where she was rummaging through her small closet packed full of clothes, purses, and shoes. I opened the freezer door before she answered. There it was. The phone was sitting on top of the ice cube tray. *How long had it been in there?*

I walked into the bedroom with the phone in hand, where my mom was on her knees, bent over, sorting through her purses, which were now piled on the bedroom floor. "Mom, I found your phone."

"Oh, I didn't know it was missing," she said as she looked up at me.

Stunned, I felt a wave of sadness. I did not have the heart to tell her that she had just been looking for it. Nor did I say where I found it.

After this discouraging exchange, I turned and walked out of the bedroom and made my way to the living room to sit for a minute. Mom took pride in her interior decorating and homemaking skills, but she had always been frugal with her purchases. While I was growing up, our formal living room was more of a showcase, albeit a very modest one. When there was money to enhance our home furnishings, Mom chose a bright Kelly green for the living room carpet. She had paid to have an old off-white couch reupholstered in a soft fabric print of flowers in green, rust, and yellow. Yet, Mom insisted on placing a plastic cover over the couch, which was removed only when we had company.

A wood stereo phonograph stood against one wall in the living room. Mom often played her favorite tunes, including country, big band, and Rat Pack albums by Dean Martin, Sammy Davis Jr., and Frank Sinatra. Whenever I hear the songs of the big band era and the twang of country western, I think fondly of Mom and her love of music. When I visited, I often played Johnny Cash albums, so we could listen to some of our favorite songs, "I Walk the Line" and "Folsom Prison Blues." Mom would smile and hum along.

We rarely spent time in the living room, except on holidays. At Christmas, Mom preferred an artificial tree. We called it "Mom's tree." It was a fake white flock tree, but in later years, she put up a silver artificial tree and sprinkled it with blue, gold, and red bulbs. We would start a fire in the brick fireplace on Christmas Eve.

Our tree, or the "kids' tree," was destined for placement in the basement recreation room, which was also our TV area. We always put up a live, scrubby green tree—not quite as sparse as the tree depicted in *A Charlie Brown Christmas*, but one with branches widely spaced. Dad would place long strings of multi-colored blinking lights on the tree, and we would decorate it with homemade ornaments, cheap, breakable bulbs, popcorn strands, and silver tinsel.

These memories, and many others, filled my thoughts whenever I returned for a visit. Mom and I would reminisce about the good and bad times. While Mom's advancing stages of short-term memory loss were increasingly apparent with each visit home, her long-term memory remained intact, allowing us to share these recollections.

Perhaps, because I saw her less frequently than my siblings and stayed with her when visiting St. Paul, I noticed things that might not have been apparent to my sisters and brothers, who did not spend the night at the house. But they were privy to other things I was not.

Mom roamed the house at night. She rarely slept and did not seem to know when it was time for bed. Although she had always been a night owl, she usually went to bed by one or two-o'clock in the morning. She had told me that while we were growing up, late night was the only time she could find peace to read, think, or watch the Johnny Carson show. This was different; she was nervous, wandering in circles and agonizing, still up at three or four in the morning.

*****

One night during another visit, I awoke to a new disturbance. I found her pacing up and down the stairs from the basement to the main floor, to the upstairs bedroom, and back down again.

"Mom, what are you doing?" I said when I woke up.

She yelled, "Where is she? Where is she? I know she is here!"

"Who are you looking for, Mom?" I inquired, still not certain what was going on. It was three in the morning.

"Sissy. Where is she?" Her anger was palpable. "She is stealing from me. I know it!" She seethed with anger.

Sissy was the youngest and had been the last to live at home with Mom. Although Dad had died when Sissy was in her first year of college, she lived at home with Mom during the summers and for a while before she married. Mom did not remember that Sissy was no longer living in her house.

"What do you mean? Sissy stealing from you? What is she stealing?" I asked, confused in the pre-dawn hour.

"She is stealing my clothes!" Mom screamed.

Trying to put some logic to the situation, I said, "Mom, Sissy is several inches taller than you and weighs more than you. Why would she steal your clothes? Your clothes won't fit her." It would never have occurred to me that Sissy would steal anything from Mom.

Her answer was immediate. "She is giving them to her friends."

"Mom, Sissy doesn't live here anymore. She married Brian a couple of years ago, and they live in Forest Lake."

I thought about what I had been reading and learning about Alzheimer's. Many people with the disease experience delusions. In other words, they hold misconceptions or false beliefs about others, often people closely related to them. The person who lives, or last lived with them, is often the target of their delusions. For example, they may accuse their spouse of cheating, or they may accuse a family member or caregiver of stealing money or precious belongings. They may also claim to actually see a person who is not there, or mistake a person for someone well-known to them.

I had just learned that you cannot reason with someone who is experiencing a delusion. These are vivid but false beliefs. In fact, if you try to argue with them, it creates more angst and may cause an escalation in what health professionals call "behaviors," such as paranoia. The best way to handle a person's delusions is to acknowledge the belief and redirect them to another activity.

Yet, here I was trying to reason with Mom. I should have said, "Mom, I will talk to Sissy about your missing clothes." When it is your loved one, though, it is difficult to understand and accept. It becomes frustrating and exhausting to constantly "be in the present" with them while avoiding arguments or showing irritation. I finally walked away from my mom and into the living room to calm myself.

There, in the living room, the cushions of Mom's favorite sofa sat high off the base of the couch. Stuffed between the cushions and the sofa foundation were layers of Mom's clothes. Visible. In plain sight. *How odd. What in the world?*

The plastic had long been removed, so we could actually go into the living room and sit without sticking to the couch like honey on bread. Unsuspecting of this spectacle, the look of distress on my face would have been noticeable to anyone—but the person having a delusion. Feeling her presence, I turned abruptly and almost bumped into Mom, who was closely trailing me.

"Mom, what are these clothes doing in here?" I was trying not to show alarm.

"I'm hiding them from Sissy," she said emphatically. Speechless, I hugged my dear, sweet mother. Then I said, "I'm sorry you are missing some of your clothes. It must be so disturbing. Now, let's go have some warm milk and graham crackers like you always suggest when I have trouble sleeping." I led her into the dining room and readied the milk and crackers. We sat in silence, sipping the warm liquid, sadness weighing heavily on my heart.

13

Love Is Not Enough

How do we keep Mom safe? The question weighed heavily as I brainstormed with my siblings during telephone calls and visits home; we were now at a crossroads, well into 1993. Thanks to the flexibility of my boss, I was in town on one of my visits to St. Paul. My siblings and I gathered at Lori's house, sharing our anxieties.

The conversation turned to me as I walked in. "Kathleen, we were discussing what to do about Mom's living situation. We don't think she can live alone much longer," Lori said. "We think you should approach her and ask if she would consider having Rodney move into her house."

Although I had been using my full name since I turned twenty, my family called me Kathi when I was growing up. Over time, my siblings became accustomed to calling me Kathleen, but Mom never did. I was always Kathi to her—and for some reason, this moment of being called Kathleen by my closest family members felt odd.

I paused for several seconds, taking in this feeling. I regressed to my childhood, seeing us all in the recreation room, playfully arguing over whose turn it was to sit in the recliner. At the same time, I was speechless by the suggestion that Rodney move in with Mom. My siblings wanted me to approach him, and everyone was on board! I was late to the discussion.

This was one of several major family meetings we had convened to commiserate over growing concerns. Our family included my siblings: Cheri, Steve, Dan, Lori, Sissy, and me. Everyone contributed ideas and support. It was rare for all of us to meet at the same time.

Often, it was just a few of us discussing action plans, then conveying the latest strategy to our other siblings.

Lori and I usually took the lead in raising an issue, especially since we were Mom's co-powers of attorney. But now, it was more important than ever that we present a united front, so everyone was there. Lori's level-headed husband, John, joined us and shared his thoughtful ideas.

John and Lori had spent a great deal of time with Mom and Dad before Dad died. After he passed away, John's carpentry skills were a godsend in helping Mom take care of her house and in working with my brothers on major home repairs, maintenance, or yard work.

Rodney lived in an apartment and took the bus to work or to meet my mom. He did not have much money, and Mom told me that she and Rodney always shared the expense of trips and outings. We had come to appreciate the time Rodney spent with Mom because we believed she was happy and safe with him. It had been nearly five years since they started seeing each other, and he always appeared to be respectful of her and courteous to us. So, we didn't pry or question his past.

We knew Rodney had five children, though we never met them, and he never spoke of his kids. When we asked Mom about it, she said he didn't like to talk about his past. Because Mom seemed to love Rodney and enjoy his company, we welcomed him unconditionally and included him in our family gatherings.

"Rodney? Move in with Mom?" My voice revealed a mix of shock and disbelief. "How did this come up? What do you mean? Let's discuss other options first."

We discussed hiring home health aides and explored the option of adult foster homes. We talked about the possibility of Mom moving north to Cheri's house, but Cheri did not embrace this option. She raised the issue of the potential for Mom to wander, reminding us that her house was surrounded by over twenty acres of wooded land.

I once contemplated the possibility of moving home to live with my mom and discussed it with her, but she was adamantly opposed to the idea. I had no illusions that I could work full-time and adequately take care of Mom in her home for the many years that she would likely live. There was no family money for long-term care at home. In the end, I gave this option little consideration because it would not be easy to find an in-house counsel job in the area, and if I worked for a law firm, I would need to take the Minnesota Bar Exam.

After weighing our options, we concluded that having Rodney move in was the most practical solution to keep Mom in her home and safe for the immediate future. We felt hopeful, yet uneasy about the decision. Based on what we knew about him, we thought he might embrace this idea, since he and Mom were spending so much time together. We devised a plan: I would be the one to approach her.

The next day, after further discussions with Lori and John, I sat down with Mom. "Mom, have you ever considered having Rodney move in with you?" I began, my heart pounding.

She looked at me with startled surprise. "I will never get married again," she stated with firm indignation. "I like my independence!"

Not expecting this reaction, I quickly blurted out, "You don't have to get married." I was secretly pleased to hear she did not want to marry Rodney. Adding a marriage to the current situation would have complicated decision-making and created possible legal issues with Mom's house and finances.

"What do you mean? What would the neighbors think if he moved in and we weren't married?" She was aghast.

"Mom, you live alone in this three-story house. If you are concerned with what the neighbors might think, you can tell them you're renting a room to Rodney. He can have the entire upstairs bedroom. You will each have independence and space. I can write up a rental agreement; after a spouse dies, many people need money. You can charge him, but not as much as he is paying for an apartment. Besides, it will help Rodney financially."

My idea to implement and execute a rental agreement with Rodney would later prove to be a blessing.

She was silent. I could see that her mind was trying to process this concept. "Mom, why don't you think about it? You don't have to decide now. Since you aren't driving anymore, you and Rodney can take the bus and go to the Manor to dance in the evenings. He won't have to take a bus or cab to come get you."

After a day of contemplation, Mom decided she liked the idea of Rodney moving in. She discussed it with him and told me he was very excited about living together. I made sure to speak with him in Mom's absence before drafting the rental agreement.

We discussed Mom's increasing memory difficulties. I told him that my siblings and I had conferred about his move into Mom's home, explaining that we were happy for them. I shared that we were appreciative that Mom could live in her home longer, and that he was willing to help keep her safe. We wanted Mom to remain independent for as long as possible. We discussed the future, and I emphasized that when Mom's needs became greater, we would have to look into moving her to a place that specialized in memory care. Rodney nodded his understanding.

We had talked with him openly about Mom's condition over the previous years, and he had accompanied her to doctor appointments. He shared his own observations with me about Mom's forgetfulness. For all practical purposes, he seemed to understand the situation and was happy to help. He also acknowledged that it was beneficial for him because we were charging less in rent than he was paying for his current apartment.

"Whatever you need, let me know. I love your mother," he said.

"Lori will come to the house several times a week to check on Mom. She will continue to bring groceries. Also, Steve, Dan, and John will continue to perform repairs on the house as needed. When you and Mom go out—or if you find yourselves splitting the price of dinner or tickets to a show—you can put the receipts in the gold cookie jar in the kitchen. Lori will reconcile expenses monthly and pay you back for Mom's half if there isn't enough money in the jar when you need it."

Rodney and I discussed safety issues and measures he could implement to keep her safe. We talked about Mom's increasing delusions and discussed some techniques he could use to distract her, such as making something to eat together or watching a show.

All was settled, and the move-in day planned. Steve, Dan, and John helped Rodney move his possessions to Mom's house. He had no issues with the rental agreement and said he was very happy to be living with Mom.

14

Intersection of Work and Personal Life

In late fall 1993, I started my dream job at the headquarters of a large national long-term care company. It took nearly six months from my first interview to the job offer because the interviewer planned to conduct a national search for someone with extensive legal experience. To overcome this, I persisted in contacting the hiring attorney, sending periodic follow-ups highlighting how my nursing experience would benefit the role and emphasizing that I was a quick learner. I even sent research papers I had written for a healthcare ethics certification course the previous year.

When the offer finally arrived that fall, I was thrilled. As Associate Counsel, I would be responsible for a wide range of legal issues in the facilities: human resources, contracts, operational advice, and regulatory appeals. Coincidentally, the corporate headquarters was located in Tacoma, directly across the street from my law school. This meant I would again be commuting nearly an hour each day from Seattle to Tacoma.

After a few days of orientation, I began on-the-job training. I immediately started receiving calls from administrators nationwide seeking legal advice. The directors of nursing contacted me about issues with residents and their families in the memory care units, also known as secure units. These specialized areas housed memory-impaired residents prone to wandering, often unaware of their surroundings.

My job was a constant reminder of Mom's increasing symptoms. Worrying about her, I called frequently. One day while at work, I could not stop thinking about her. I picked up the phone and called.

"Hello," her voice sounded like a soft whisper.

"Hi, Mom," I said.

"Oh, I'm so glad to hear your voice! I'm scared. I locked Sissy in the shed three days ago, and I think she's still in there. I was so mad at her for taking my clothes, but she hasn't had any food or water for three days. I'm too scared to go out there."

Panic colored her voice. Mom's house was connected to a screened-in porch with a shed in the back, where she stored the bikes, the lawnmower, and her gardening tools. It took me a moment to absorb her words. Then it occurred to me that this was another delusion. *What should I say?*

"Oh, oh, hi Steve!" I heard her excited voice trail off as she turned away from the telephone receiver. She was always so happy to see my brother.

Steve worked as a roofer for the St. Paul School District. He often stopped in to see Mom between jobs. I considered it a blessing that he could visit her during the day, several times a week, and he was grateful his job gave him the flexibility to check on her.

"Mom," I raised my voice so she would put the receiver back to her ear. "Mom, please put Steve on the phone."

After she handed the phone to Steve, I said, "Steve, I just happened to call Mom. It sounds like she is in a panic. She believes she locked Sissy in the shed three days ago. Would you tell her you'll go out and look in the shed to see if Sissy is still locked in? I think this is another one of her delusions." I paused to see if he had any questions.

"I see," he said, realizing Mom was listening intently. "Yes, I will check." He didn't ask anything more, fully aware of the pattern of Mom's recent delusions. He gave the phone back to Mom and told her he would go out to check on Sissy.

Steve walked out the kitchen door and through the porch to the shed. Mom was back on the phone, talking to me. I could tell she was looking out the open kitchen window into the porch. She was watching him. She talked hesitantly into the phone, "Oh, I'm so glad he stopped by. He's opening the door now to see if Sissy is still there," she reported. There was a long pause. "Oh, good!" she whispered with relief into the phone. "He is shaking his head no."

"No, Mom, Sissy must have gotten out. She is not in the shed," Steve stated loudly, so I could hear through the telephone receiver.

"Oh, thank goodness," she said with relief. "I was so worried. But you know how mad I get at her."

Once he was back in the house, he took the phone from Mom while asking her if Rodney was at home. I heard her say he was at work. Steve spoke into the receiver, "Hi, Kath, I'll stay and visit with Mom for a while before I head back to work; Rodney's not here."

"Thanks, Steve. Sometimes it's so frustrating being so far away. I'm so grateful that you're able to stop by to check on Mom during your busy work days." I hung up, sighing with relief.

Sitting alone in my office, I was thankful no one witnessed the tears in my eyes. Even with Rodney living at the house, we remained ever vigilant. It takes all of us working together to support Mom. I was thankful for my siblings.

15

Attempts at Creating Routine

Rodney had his own refuge upstairs in what we had called the "girls'" bedroom for most of our lives. However, I suspected he didn't often spend the entire night up there.

Whenever I was in town, I stayed in Steve and Dan's former bedroom, just down the hall from Mom. Rodney would retreat upstairs, but he usually fell asleep first in the recreation room where he and Mom watched TV. This routine gave me a strange feeling—it had been Dad's habit to fall asleep downstairs. Despite these shifting dynamics, visiting intermittently allowed me to accurately assess Mom's condition and coping skills around the clock.

As the winter of 1994 arrived, we were gradually becoming more comfortable with the new living arrangement. Rodney was at home with Mom much of the day and able to keep an eye on her for immediate dangers. Mom was still physically able to take care of her own personal bathing and dressing needs, although it took her longer. When visiting that winter, I found myself having to prompt her more frequently when she was dressing or applying her makeup. It became evident that she was experiencing an inability to stay focused.

Despite taking more time to complete tasks, she was still able to walk and get around, even with her increasing periods of confusion. Rodney and Mom continued to go out dancing or to a movie. Her level of awareness and fear appeared to keep her from aimless wandering, a condition that can affect people at various stages of dementia; it is different for each individual.

We hired Candy, a home health aide, to stay with Mom when Rodney was at work. He wanted to quit his job and stay home with her, but we advised him to continue working. We did not want him to be totally burdened with caregiving and knew he needed his own money. Between family and hired help, we made sure Mom was never alone.

In early 1994, Mom needed surgery for a hernia repair. Lori scheduled the surgery, and Cheri was able to drive down to the Twin Cities to help with Mom's recovery. Lori continued frequent visits to Mom's home, dropping off groceries and other necessities. If she left the house when Rodney was going to work, she offered to drive him to the bus. During these months, I recognized how much Lori and John did for Mom on a routine basis and was so appreciative that they were local. While long-distance caregiving can be difficult and frustrating, I did as much as I could. I did my best to address issues over the phone, sending letters to her, and planning visits back home.

In a letter to Lori in January that year, I discussed issues such as Mom's taxes, Rodney's rent money, and other concerns. I also wrote: "Once again, thank you for all your work and efforts on behalf of our dear mother. I only wish things were different and we didn't have to deal with this. I think it is very important that you take care of yourself and your family as well. Please call and talk to me whenever you are feeling overwhelmed, and we can continue to brainstorm on possible care options."

Family members often don't know or appreciate the expenses incurred by the long-distance caregiver, such as traveling or taking time off work without pay when necessary. Before cell phones, the telephone charges were also significant. As a family, it is vital to communicate effectively and to work together. It is essential to appreciate and incorporate the unique contributions of each family member in the caregiving process.

Because my job required travel, I took advantage of combining my business trips with stopovers in Minnesota, using my vacation days. My boss continued to be understanding of these issues. Working for a national long-term care company had its advantages.

Whenever I knew in advance that I would be in Minnesota for a few days, I suggested that Lori schedule medical appointments for

Mom during this window, so I could help lessen some of her burden. I hoped that these opportunities would provide a brief respite for Lori and tried to give her as much notice as possible so she could take advantage of my presence. I know Dan helped get Mom to her appointments when he was available.

Everyone tried to help, but it was not an easy task. All my brothers and sisters were raising families and working, or had family concerns of their own to deal with. Steve's frequent visits to check on Mom during the work week abruptly ended in December 1994 when he had his own major medical problems to contend with.

Sissy was unable to help in person because of Mom's paranoia towards her. Mom's delusions were getting worse, and on one occasion, she told me she put a baseball bat by the door to keep Sissy away. "I know she is my daughter," she said emphatically, "but I don't want her here. I will scare her away with this bat if she tries to come in."

My heart went out to Sissy. She was only eighteen when Dad died. Now she was being rejected and essentially banned from being alone with Mom. For some reason, when we were all together at a large gathering, Mom's delusions about Sissy didn't manifest in the same way. I was thankful, though, that Sissy was married to a great guy and had a wonderful mother-in-law.

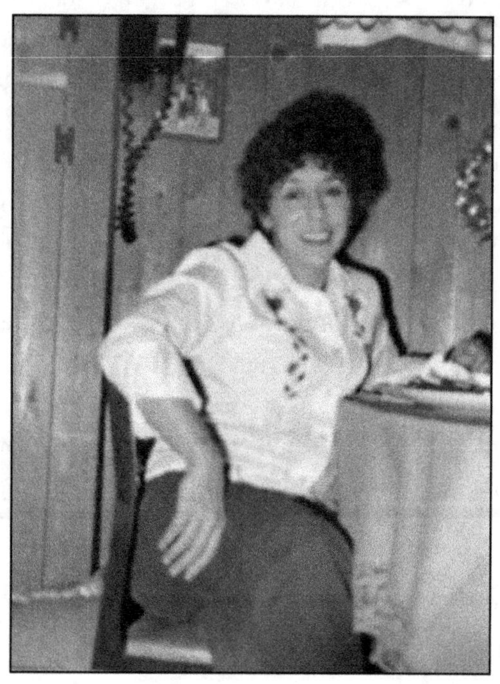

Mom in the recreation room

16

Annual Thanksgiving Holidays

Turkey or no turkey?

When I think about Thanksgiving, I recall happy family gatherings and time alone with Mom, but also sad memories of her decline. Typically, my siblings were busy with their own family traditions and in-law visits during the Christmas holidays, so I chose the Thanksgiving weekend as my time to visit Minnesota. This allowed time with my mom and visits with my siblings and their families. Visiting in November also allowed me to avoid the sometimes-harsh December weather in Minnesota.

When Dad died in 1987, I went home for Christmas. After that, knowing Mom had Rodney around during the holidays eased my guilt in not being home in December. But every Thanksgiving weekend, I stayed at my mom's house and helped her host the family's annual turkey dinner.

She loved the tradition of shopping on Black Friday, so we continued this practice each year. We would shop for all my siblings and Mom's grandchildren. We wrapped the gifts and put them in the closet before the weekend was over, ready for Lori to deliver to everyone at Christmas time.

Mom's favorite place to shop when we were growing up was a shopping center in West St. Paul called Signal Hills. When the Mall of America opened in Minneapolis in 1992, it was a new and novel attraction in Minnesota. In the years after its grand opening, we would shop there often, even if it wasn't Black Friday.

If we were at the Mall of America, Mom's pace would pick up when she spotted the Cinnabon store, taking in the familiar smell of spicy cinnamon. She clearly remembered the sweet taste of the glazed frosting, too. We would buy one to split and sit with a cup of coffee, savoring the warmth of the food and drink.

While her memories of food and taste stayed with her for years, her fear of getting lost increased. She was more cautious and scared and stayed closer to me when we went shopping. I would keep a watchful eye on her while I rifled through the racks at Nordstrom's.

"Kathi, Kathi, where are you?" If she lost sight of me, she yelled my name as she stood in place, frightened and wide-eyed, her head shifting back and forth.

"Mom, I'm right here," I shouted as I rushed to her side.

During the Thanksgiving holidays in 1993, I invited Lori's daughter, my niece Andrea, to join my mom and me on one of our traditional trips to the Mall. Andrea, a sweet, dark-eyed beauty, loved her grandmother, but at eight years old, she didn't understand her periods of confusion. She once asked me if we would all be happier if Grandma weren't sick.

The Mall of America is a massive multilevel structure that boasts a movie theater, food court, and indoor amusement center—one of the unique ideas that brought it fame. Bustling with holiday activity and beautiful Christmas decorations, Andrea bubbled with enthusiasm, especially as we approached the indoor Ferris wheel.

"Auntie! Auntie! Can we go on the rides?" she pleaded.

I turned to face Mom. "Mom, will you be okay standing here while Andrea and I go on the Ferris wheel? Will you please wait right here?" I was hesitant because I had heard stories about people with dementia wandering off at shopping malls and getting lost, only to be found too late. This concern played frequently in my mind. I pushed these thoughts aside. Thank goodness, Mom still had the fear of getting lost and didn't yet wander aimlessly.

"Mom, if I take Andrea on the Ferris wheel, will you wait right here for us?" I repeated, making sure she understood. "You can watch us from here." I pointed to the looming wheels circling in the air.

"Yes," she answered confidently.

I took a chance, and Andrea and I went on the ride. I strained to see Mom the whole time, torn between enjoying my time with my niece and watching her. After the ride, Andrea and I hurried back to Mom, where she stood steadfastly gazing at her surroundings—in the exact spot where we left her. Relief flooded through me. Andrea and I did not go on any more rides that day.

*****

Work issues prevented me from traveling home for Thanksgiving in 1994. As I often did on holidays when not in town, I called Mom's house late in the afternoon. Dinner would be over, and everyone would be watching TV or playing games. Lori answered.

"Happy Thanksgiving!" I cheered. "I assume you're all done with dinner?"

"No, John just arrived with the Kentucky Fried Chicken," Lori said with a sigh.

"What?" I exclaimed.

"We're having Kentucky Fried Chicken," Lori said with a heaviness in her voice. "Mom put the turkey in the oven early this morning, but forgot to turn it on."

I was stunned. "What? Didn't she check it periodically?"

"No one was paying much attention. I bought the turkey and took it over to Mom's house a few days ago. I know Mom has a difficult time focusing on cooking, but Rodney said he knew how to make a turkey, and he would work with Mom to get it in the oven on Thanksgiving morning. None of us really paid attention until John said, 'Lori, I don't smell the turkey. Usually, we can smell it by now.'"

Lori continued, "I ran upstairs to the kitchen, opened the oven, and saw the pale twenty-pound turkey. Raw. By that time, we were all very hungry, so John volunteered to go get chicken.

"Mom feels really bad one minute, but then she doesn't seem to recall that it's Thanksgiving Day. You know how she enjoys Kentucky Fried Chicken. And of course, we have her favorite coleslaw from Cecil's Delicatessen, and I made the mashed potatoes

91

and stuffing. Sissy and Brian brought side dishes, and Cheri brought the pies. So, I guess it'll all work out."

Lori lamented the fact that she didn't pay more attention that day. The turkey had already been in the oven when she arrived with John and the kids. Down in the "rec room," Lori got caught up visiting with Dan and his fiancée, Lynn, who arrived shortly after her. They were there for a short visit before going to Lynn's mother's home.

Mom still had periodic times of lucidity. In her own home with loved ones around, it was easier to fall into old routines and patterns, and not supervise her every minute, believing she could still live a normal life. Denial is a powerful psychological defense; it allowed us to trust she could manage. Also, in previous years, because I was home for Thanksgiving and staying at Mom's, I was there helping prepare the feast with Mom in the kitchen, making sure everything stayed on track.

Part IV

A Tumultuous Year: 1995

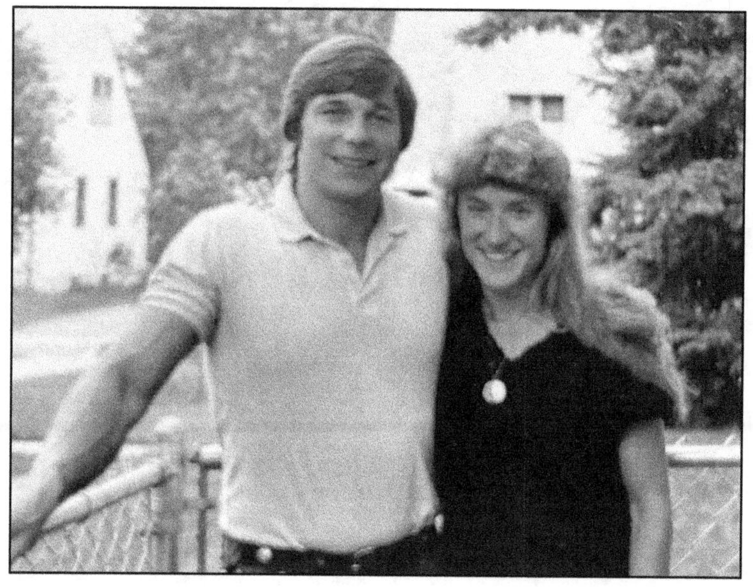

Steve and Kathleen: Labor Day Weekend 1986

17

Steve's Medical Crisis

After hearing about the Thanksgiving incident and then learning from Lori about Rodney's disturbing behavior toward her, a sense of dismay consumed me. It was difficult to digest that Rodney had been making passes at Lori, and she did not share it with me sooner. Most important, it was painfully clear that my mom's condition was deteriorating faster than I had expected, and we could no longer rely on Rodney. We urgently needed to find her a safe place to live.

As the cold, icy days of the impending holiday season shortened and darkness descended, one crisis followed another. The already difficult search for a new place for Mom was interrupted when my brother Steve was hospitalized for emergency brain surgery.

Earlier that year, nine months before his December medical crisis, Steve called to tell me he was experiencing double vision, difficulty walking, and recurring falls. This was particularly distressing because his job involved roof installations and repairs. He insisted he wasn't drinking or using drugs, which I believed. Although Steve had struggled with alcohol use, in recent years, he had adopted a healthier lifestyle, spending time with his children and frequently visiting Mom to ensure her safety.

After discussing his symptoms in the spring, I advised him to consult a neurologist. Following several doctors' appointments, Steve was diagnosed with hydrocephalus, a condition where the brain is unable to properly drain cerebrospinal fluid, leading to a buildup. The doctors were unclear as to what caused his initial crisis, but suspected it was a minor birth defect, a stenosis—or narrowing of the brain's ventricles. Over many years, the narrowing led to the accumulation of excess fluid, which caused his symptoms, including headaches, blurred vision, balance problems, and short-term memory deficit.

His treatment started in April 1994 with the surgical placement of a shunt—a flexible tube—into his brain to divert the accumulated fluid to the peritoneal cavity (the space in the abdomen that holds organs). After the initial placement, Steve required subsequent surgeries to replace infected shunts. The doctors explained that problems with shunt adjustments and infections were not unusual at his age of thirty-nine, because the body needs time to adjust to a foreign object.

Steve kept me informed of his medical issues over the year, and I discussed his condition with Mom, trying to alleviate any angst she was having about his health.

In early December, while recovering from a hernia surgery at home, Steve became delirious. He spoke to his wife as if he were still stationed in Germany twenty years earlier. She rushed him to the hospital. Over the next three weeks, he endured several brain surgeries to replace an infected shunt, and then slipped into a coma.

Once I learned about Steve's condition, I made plans to travel to Minnesota and took a leave of absence from my job until mid-January. Over the holidays and into the new year, Steve's wife and children, my siblings, and I waited long hours at the hospital. We rotated periodically, so someone was either by his side or in the waiting area of the intensive care unit (ICU). We were allowed to visit him, one person at a time, for short periods.

The nurses and doctors prepared us for the worst, telling us to plan for his passing. When we stood by his bedside, the constant beeping of the machines was disturbing, and the rushing around of medical staff disconcerting. I had worked in a pediatric ICU at Seattle Children's Hospital, so I was familiar with the chaotic environment and distress of family members.

Despite my experience, it is different when it is someone you know and love. As a family member, I searched the faces of his nurses and doctors, asking questions that prompted honest discussions. One morning, Steve's wife expressed concerns that the nurses and doctors were no longer as attentive to him once they thought he might die. I could not disagree.

Meanwhile, at home, my mother was anxious and agitated, telling me over dinner that she wanted to be at the hospital with Steve. Although she was sometimes lucid enough to remember he was in the hospital, when I called the house to check on her during the day, she had often forgotten that he was ill. Candy, Mom's home health aide, stayed with her every day Rodney worked, ensuring she was never alone.

Due to her growing needs, Mom required constant supervision. Taking her to the hospital would have heightened her agitation significantly. The flurry of activity when the doors opened into the ICU, the anxiety of other families, and most importantly, the uncertainty of Steve's recovery would have overwhelmed her. Mom had lost some of her inhibitions about wandering, so we had to watch her closely when we took her out. Yet, I struggled with whether I should take her to the hospital. I felt she needed to see Steve at least one more time if he was going to die.

Mom loved all her children. Although I cannot speak for my other siblings, I always believed that Mom and Dad loved and treated their children equally, giving to each of us according to our individual needs. Yet, I believed there was a special bond with Mom and her sons. Steve was especially sensitive; Mom sensed this. He looked after her as she did him.

Steve adored our dad and would fish and hunt with him, but I knew Dad's drinking troubled him when we were growing up. Like me, he saw how sad it made Mom. He reacted by experimenting with smoking cigarettes and marijuana, drinking, and skipping school. Dad was furious with Steve's reckless behavior; his reaction was akin to "do as I say, not as I do."

While Steve and I attended different high schools and had separate circles of friends, we stayed connected because we were only fourteen months apart in age. During high school, Steve would often invite me to parties with him, where we both knew there would be drinking.

Sometimes I accompanied him, but he was always respectful if I said no. When I was fifteen, I agreed to smoke a cigarette with him—once.

When Steve was a junior in high school, Dad pressured him to enlist in the Army. His rationale was that it "would make a man out of him." But he was too young to enlist without a parent's signature. So, when Steve turned seventeen in February of 1972, Dad signed for him—and off he went in the spring to join the U.S. Army. Mom told me then that she didn't think she could ever forgive Dad for sending Steve away.

After he left home, we communicated through handwritten letters. Months before my graduation from high school in 1974, my brother's letters became more enthusiastic than those of the previous year. They were filled with enticing ideas about what we could do together if I lived and traveled in Europe for a year. I did some research and decided to defer going to college. My plan was to live in the same town where Steve was stationed; he said it would be easy for me to get a job on base in the post exchange store or as a waitress in the officers' club. We planned to explore Europe in the spring of 1975, following his discharge from the Army.

Distressingly, three weeks before I left that summer, I received a letter from my brother with jarring news. Mom had gotten the mail that day and handed me the envelope. As always, when one of us heard from him, we waited by each other's side to hear his news. Mom saw my eyes moisten as I read the letter. "What is it?" She was visibly anxious.

In his letter, Steve asked me not to tell Mom or Dad that he had been arrested for possession of hashish. But Mom was right there as I read his words. When she saw the tears streaming down my face, she grabbed the paper from my hands. I cried out that Steve had been arrested. "He's in the U.S. Army prison in Mannheim, Mom!"

Now, with his admission in hand, Mom began to read. Stunned, angry, and sad all at once, she tried to stifle her cries. After finishing the letter, she hurried to the phone to make some calls to see if she could initiate help for Steve. After I had time to absorb the news and reread his account, I decided to continue with my plans. Steve had given me the name of a friend to contact who would help me get settled during my first weeks in Germany.

When I left in June 1974, I went straight to a small town called Viernheim so I could be near the Mannheim Military Prison. The only approved visiting days were on weekends and holidays. Each time I arrived at the formidable prison grounds, I was processed in, always with the threat of being patted down and fully searched. Then, I was taken to the large visiting room where the guards watched everyone closely. A sense of melancholy lingered within me as I visited with my brother. I surveyed the visitors' room, observing so many young men. Their youth made the confinement so much more poignant. During our lengthy talks and some prayer time, Steve shared that he was involved in prison Bible studies, which gave him comfort and helped him get through each day.

After our visit, he was led to a solitary room where he had to undress so the guards could examine him to make sure I didn't secretly give him anything—not even a picture. Then, he could return to his cell.

Steve spent just over a month in Mannheim before being transferred to Leavenworth, Kansas, where he served about six months. As a non-violent inmate, he was assigned to the satellite federal prison camp. I don't think he could ever intentionally hurt anyone; he has a tender heart and treats people kindly. Steve finished his sentence under minimum security, spending time outdoors while working on the prison farm, an assignment for which he told me he was grateful.

Steve and I both wrote long, frequent letters to Mom—him from prison and me from my travel destinations. She was heartsick about his incarceration and constantly concerned for his safety. It wasn't until years later that I learned how encumbered with worry she also was regarding my wellbeing as I traveled alone throughout Europe and Israel—despite her outward support for my new adventures.

I kept both Mom and Steve apprised of my whereabouts, and they would send letters to me in care of the American Express office in each city I visited. I still remember the anticipation of picking up a letter from family or friends after traveling alone to a new town. These offices were also helpful for making travel reservations and providing assistance in case of emergencies, which gave Mom a sense of comfort.

In her letters, Mom made it clear how much she cherished the news I sent her and the letters she received from Steve. While she was grateful that Steve's strong faith sustained him, she was frustrated that he so often quoted the Bible and talked of Jesus' teachings, page after page. Once, when I was on a rare telephone call with Mom from overseas, she lamented, "Steve's letters are filled with quotes from the Bible. I want to hear about him, how he is really coping. His letters are more preachy than newsy. I worry about him," she said. I understood because I received the same type of letters from him. However, I was encouraged by his faith, which reinforced mine as I traveled and hitchhiked alone.

Steve had spent over two and a half years in the military, much of it in the 8th Infantry Division, participating in tank training missions in Baumholder. He sustained an unblemished record, receiving accolades for his work in the infantry, including an award as the best tank driver. Ultimately, Steve appealed his conviction and succeeded in getting it overturned, and in due course, received a general discharge under honorable conditions. Mom was elated when she heard.

*****

On January 13, 1995, I received a call from Sissy while at Mom's house. Her excitement caught me off guard. "Kath, Brian and I were visiting Steve early this morning. Sometimes we go and pray over him. While I was looking down at him in bed, he opened his eyes. He woke up from his coma! He looked at me and moved his eyes. I called out for the nurse to come in. Kath, Steve is awake!"

After several weeks in a coma, Steve was awake and alert, but the rest of his body was still paralyzed. I told Mom the good news, and we visited him the next day. Over the course of a week, Steve's body slowly came to life. First, he moved his head from side to side, then raised his arms; finally, he lifted and moved his legs.

Steve tells an amazing story about how, when he was in his coma trying to transition to the other side, Dad came to him and told him to go back, that it wasn't his time yet. Once, I made the mistake of calling his story a dream. He immediately corrected me.

"No, Sister! It was not a dream. Dad was there. He came to tell me that I wasn't done on this earth yet." His certainty about his spiritual experience left me contemplating the mysterious nature of such encounters. To this day, Steve's faith leads him. He continues to share his life's story and approves of me writing about him.

During the year of his rehabilitation, significant changes took place for all of us, including the sale of our family home.

18

A Bad Situation

Lori continued to emphasize the need to find a place for Mom. Once Steve awoke from his coma and his immediate medical crisis abated, we were able to return our focus to the search. While we were fortunate to have several home health aides stay with Mom when Rodney was out, his living at the house was causing Lori angst. She often encountered him during her frequent visits.

She had finally shared that during the previous summer and fall, Rodney had declared his love for her. Not to Mom, but to Lori! *What?* She said she was at her "wits' end" with him.

Lori didn't tell me about these declarations when they happened. Nor did she tell me about the first "love note" he wrote to her. But after she received the second letter in late fall of 1994, intensifying her worry, she shared these shocking incidents of Rodney's advances. When she related the information to me long after the first event, she tried to describe how Rodney had confided in her about his feelings. "Kath, you wouldn't believe the things he said to me." Lori's distressed voice had my attention.

She paraphrased his words: "Lori, don't you remember when you looked into my eyes on Thanksgiving last year and gave me a big hug? And when you rubbed against me when we passed each other in the hallway at the house last month? I know you have feelings for me, too."

Lori said she was stunned at his revelations. "Rodney," she had said, showing her alarm, "I am married. Married. I have a husband. I love my husband. What are you talking about? If I gave you a hug, it's because you're part of our family. We hug each other. We're an affectionate family. What are you talking about when you say 'I rubbed up against you'? I come to the house often. I was probably rushing past you in a hurry—as often happens when I come to check on Mom. I have a family and two young children. What're you thinking? I thought you loved my mom?"

Rodney didn't seem to understand the implications of his confession. For Lori, the primary fear was that Mom's comfort and safety would be threatened by Rodney's inappropriate behavior. After she confided in me, we had several contemplative phone calls. We decided not to immediately address the issue with either Rodney or Mom. We couldn't predict their reactions, and we didn't want to alienate or distress Mom if she didn't believe us. Her current delusions were already concerning. Not knowing how to best protect Mom without alienating her was a driving concern.

We needed a plan. I advised Lori to keep the notes in a safe place in case they became important in the future. Later, it would prove to be a wise decision.

Lori was no longer comfortable going to Mom's house with Rodney's continued inappropriate overtures. The Thanksgiving event became clearer to me as I reflected on it. Rodney said he would help Mom make the turkey, and Lori tried to avoid him as much as she could while at Mom's house.

Increasingly upset and in crisis mode, Lori was adamant that we needed to make plans to move Mom into an adult foster care or nursing home situation. She did not have the patience to continue to put up with Rodney's deceptive behavior. I did not blame her. I knew I had to help.

We discussed Rodney's actions and tried to make a dire situation lighthearted. He, too, must be delusional. What was his problem or issue? Perhaps he was a concrete thinker and couldn't assimilate Lori's normal generosity in driving him to the bus stop or to work when he was leaving the house at the same time. He didn't seem to understand that she was affectionate and kind to everyone. We realized how little we knew him.

We had trusted Mom's judgment and wanted her to be happy. We knew that she had had a long-time relationship with Juanita, who was both Rodney's sister and her high school friend. Thus, we didn't think of Rodney as a stranger to Mom. However, Rodney's behavior now gave us grave concern. Mom was a vulnerable adult. At this point, I wasn't really concerned that Rodney would physically harm Mom since I had spent much time in his presence, in Mexico, and when they came to visit me in Seattle. Additionally, whenever I visited Minnesota, I stayed at the house.

John, Lori's husband, sat down with Rodney one day to remind him that Lori was his wife and that he needed to stay away from her. "Rodney, Lori is my wife, and I expect you to respect that," John said firmly and directly.

Trying to rationalize this unacceptable behavior, I thought Rodney was likely moving through his own grieving process of losing Mom piece by piece. Of my three sisters, Lori most resembles my mom, with her dark brown eyes, dark hair, and olive skin. And, of course, Lori was a frequent presence in their lives.

Still trying to make sense of these revelations—which I learned about just before Steve's December hospitalization—my mind raced back to all the time I had spent with Rodney and Mom. Did I miss something? What do we do now? Should we discuss this with Mom? Devastate her? What would be in her best interests? What should our next steps be?

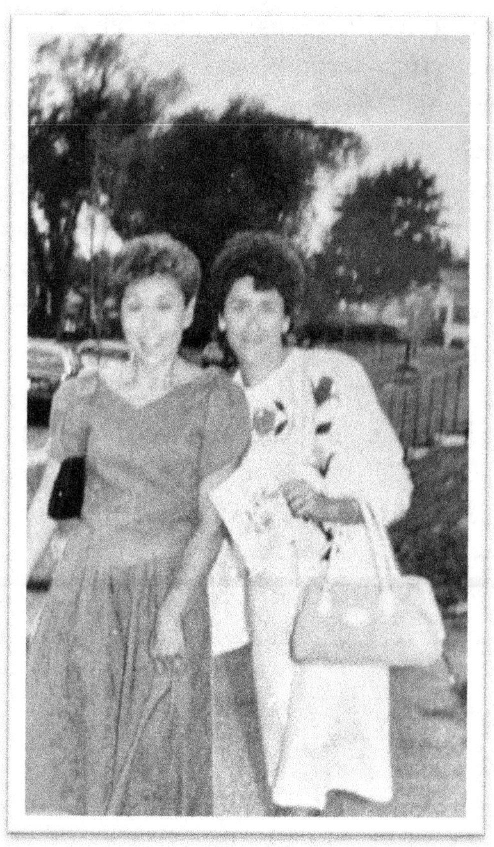

Mom and Lori

19

Looking for Placement

In January, my siblings and I discussed options for Mom as we sat at Ramsey Hospital waiting for news about Steve. Our nerves were frayed as we tried to talk under the bright lights in the waiting room of the intensive care unit. Every time a doctor or nurse opened the doors to approach tearful family members with updates, the loud, unforgiving beeps of high-tech machines followed them. We finally agreed to meet at Lori's house. All my siblings would be there except, of course, Steve, who was painfully absent.

We were devastated, not knowing what the future held for him. Adding to our grief, we were tasked with moving Mom. One night at dinner, as I updated her on Steve, she interrupted me to ask a question, but stopped mid-sentence. Her eyes clouded over. She took another bite of salad and looked at me with a blank stare. A few moments later, she asked me how Steve was doing. It was a heartbreaking reminder that we were losing her, deepening my sense of anguish. While it was difficult to accept, it was clear that she required more direct, intentional, and vigilant care.

Two days later, sitting in Lori's living room, we discussed adult foster home options and memory care units. This conversation marked our family's first real exploration of alternative living arrangements. Though a nursing facility would likely be needed as her disease advanced, we were not prepared to make that decision. Mom still had lucid moments, and the thought that she would be aware of having to leave her home was heartbreaking, especially if it meant a move to a facility.

I started having trouble sleeping and would wake up from a recurring nightmare where I was facing Mom, who was crying and screaming at me, "Promise me, Kathi, no nursing home! I want to stay in my own home!"

Circumstantial depression pulled me down into the depths of despair. Seeing no other options, I made appointments at several places in the Twin Cities—licensed, private-pay facilities and Medicare-and Medicaid-certified homes. I tried to envision my mom and my brother in the various facilities. Since Steve would need extensive rehab, his wife welcomed the idea that we also look at places with him in mind.

When entering a nursing facility, I requested copies of their most recent annual inspection and complaint survey reports from the past year. These documents provide a wealth of information about potential problems the facility may have encountered in complying with the Centers for Medicare & Medicaid Services' (CMS) regulations governing the safety of the homes and the quality of the care provided. Payments made to certified facilities are contingent upon their compliance with CMS regulations, which require that all CMS-certified facilities be inspected annually or upon receipt of a complaint. The surveys are usually conducted by the state department of health on behalf of CMS. The final written reports must be made available on the premises. Today, the results are also available online at Medicare.gov.

In addition to the survey results, in 2008, Medicare introduced a Five-Star Quality Rating System to help consumers select and compare skilled nursing care centers. Factors that contribute to achieving a five-star status include health inspection and surveys, quality care measures, and staffing. It is not a foolproof system, but it works as a guide to finding a home, just as we review star ratings for hotels and restaurants. This information is also online on the CMS website.

As we weighed these reports and compared facilities, we also researched alternatives to nursing homes. We found an adult foster care situation that we thought might be a good fit for Mom. These places are generally smaller homes licensed by the state, although some states categorize them as assisted living. Assisted living is usually a higher level of care and is governed by state regulations. Nursing facilities, which provide advanced care at a higher skill level, require a state license to operate *and* a federal CMS certification in order to bill Medicare or Medicaid.

Lori heard of Hope House, a licensed adult foster care home, where five to eight people with Alzheimer's disease lived together, like family. At least that is what I wanted to believe. Hope House had existed since 1990. Residents were cared for by home care aides who were specially trained in working with individuals with memory impairments. The mission statement read: "We promote dignity in the care of the individuals living with memory loss in a loving home environment."

Hope House was located less than a mile from the home of my Aunt Gussie, Mom's sister. Gussie, thirteen years older than Mom, lived independently and maintained an active social life despite not driving. We knew that if Mom was living at Hope House, my aunt would surely visit her.

Lori and I visited the home. We discussed taking Mom, but we wanted to see the place first to determine if it was a viable option. During our tour, we were hopeful. While the home's layout was concerning—specifically a staircase some residents had to navigate— the atmosphere appeared to be one of cooperation. Mom was still able to walk and navigate stairs, but for how long I wondered. I had already visited several larger facilities in the Twin Cities and did not feel it was the right time for Mom to be placed in one of them. I desperately wanted this place to be our answer.

Even though it was difficult, we had already engaged Mom in discussions about moving. We hoped she might like living in this home. In particular, we had the notion that she would enjoy helping people there, and if she thought of herself as a caregiver, she might be more receptive to the idea. Perhaps it was wishful thinking—but we were desperate.

We continued our discussions about Rodney's abhorrent behavior, but decided that telling Mom about his indiscretions would be cruel. What ethical actions should we take, if any, and how? We were conflicted. Given Mom's paranoia and delusional behaviors, we thought she might actually believe we were fabricating these stories. The only thing we knew for certain was that we could not allow Rodney to stay with her much longer.

During my stays at Mom's house, I often heard Rodney snap at her. Sometimes his comments were unkind. Even though Mom quickly forgot what he said, I realized this could be considered a form of emotional abuse. Caring for someone with memory loss is hard, and making a mean comment or shouting at them happens. But Lori and I now realized that something was not quite right with Rodney—especially since he didn't seem to understand the seriousness of his actions. He also told Lori that he and Mom hadn't been close physically for some time. While I didn't believe he would physically harm her, we had to consider the possibility that he might be forceful.

At work, I was dealing with situations in nursing homes where some Alzheimer's residents were sexually uninhibited. On occasions, men and women were found by the staff in their rooms engaging in sexual activity, which could then create legal issues for the facilities because of informed consent and concern for visiting spouses. While lack of sexual constraint is not always a characteristic of Alzheimer's, I did keep this in mind as we looked for placement. Some facilities had secure units for females only, and I liked the idea of placing Mom in one, if possible.

When we first approached Rodney about living with Mom, Rodney and I had had a frank discussion about the Alzheimer's disease process—the inevitable mental and physical deterioration. We had discussed that at some time in the future, we would have to move Mom to a place with specialized care for memory-impaired people, and at that time, we would sell the house. Rodney was accepting of this back then.

Meanwhile, he had become quite comfortable with his living arrangement at Mom's house. He now seemed resistant to the idea of moving Mom, which would ultimately mean he would be forced to leave the house as well. In retrospect, I was relieved we had a formal lease agreement. I had the distinct feeling it would be difficult to get him to agree to move.

Kathleen A. Hessler

20

Devastating Diagnosis and Denial

Mom had the classic symptoms of Alzheimer's disease. We experienced it—her memory loss, the delusions and paranoia, and the slow loss of physical abilities. We received confirmation from her physicians that she was suffering from memory loss, *likely* Alzheimer's.

In the 1990s, many physicians were reluctant to definitively diagnose memory loss as Alzheimer's because diagnostic tools were limited to clinical observation and cognitive testing. Today, more advanced tests are available that can help confirm a diagnosis; however, these tests also require ruling out other causes of memory loss.

After nearly six years of observing Mom's slow decline, I continued to struggle with the finality of this diagnosis in someone so young. She was fifty-nine now. The thought of her absolute decline overwhelmed me, especially after learning more about the disease.

In my job as an attorney in long-term care, I was living and breathing the life inside nursing homes, the residents' issues, and family turmoil. One could say that I had been on a fast track in 1994 for learning about memory problems, the dementia process, and how residents and families cope. Additionally, I learned that there are other medical reasons for memory loss, some of which may be reversible.

Currently, doctors typically make a presumptive diagnosis of Alzheimer's by reviewing the patient's medical history, conducting a physical examination, administering neurological tests, and using cognitive assessments to evaluate memory and thinking. Also, today blood tests are available that measure beta-amyloid and tau protein levels, which aid in diagnosing and staging the disease. One such test, called Lumipulse, received FDA approval in 2025.

Additionally, imaging tests such as CT, MRI, or PET scans are used to help rule out other medical causes of memory loss. These include: transient ischemic attack (TIA or mini-stroke), major stroke, brain hemorrhage, or hydrocephalus (a condition like my brother Steve experienced). CT and MRI scans provide visual images of the brain's physical structure, while PET scans show visual images of the brain's functional activity, which can aid in the diagnosis of Alzheimer's. The scans may also reveal shrinkage in specific parts of the brain, a sign that may indicate aging.

Scans are expensive, and some physicians may be reluctant to order them unless they are critically indicated. Because Mom was only in her early fifties when her symptoms started, I wanted to know the etiology of her memory issues with greater certainty. Now that I had a better understanding of how imaging tests can aid in the diagnosis of Alzheimer's, I wanted Mom to have an MRI, which no physician had previously ordered. (PET scans were not yet widely used for aiding in the diagnosis of Alzheimer's.)

I also knew there were medications that might help alleviate Mom's progressive suffering from agitation, paranoia, and delusions. The delusions were increasing, escalating to episodes of extreme anger and belligerence. On one recent occasion, Lori went to the house to drop off groceries while Rodney was at work. The home health aide had left early that day. Lori opened the door, and several knives fell to the floor.

"Mom," Lori called out, "what are these knives doing in the door?"

Mom rushed into the kitchen and was quick to reply. "I know Sissy is trying to get in, and I want to be ready. I don't want to hurt her, but I want her to know that I will not tolerate her coming into my house and stealing from me."

Through my research, I learned about Dr. Kay, a well-respected neurologist who had the authority to order an MRI. He could also evaluate Mom for prescriptions to help manage or alleviate her delusions and risky behaviors. I had read about experimental drug trials for patients in various stages of Alzheimer's; while I didn't know much about these studies, I was certain the neurologist would be familiar with the latest research. Once I knew I would be in Minnesota in January 1995 to visit Steve at the hospital, I made an appointment for Mom to see Dr. Kay at the University of Minnesota.

On the day of her appointment, I talked with her before we left the house, gently explaining that I was going to ask the doctor to order an MRI and medications to help her feel better.

"Oh, Kathi, do you really think this doctor will be able to help me?" Mom asked as we were getting ready to walk out the door.

"I hope so, Mom," I replied with an ache in my heart, looking at her before I opened the door.

"Me too. I would feel so much better if this doctor could help me." She reached over to hug me.

It was a cold January day. Gray overcast shed its dreariness across the city and settled into my being. We drove in silence much of the way. Mom's nervousness was overcome by hope that passed over into oblivion and delusional talk one minute, only to return to lucidity the next. It was an odd mixture of truth and fiction.

We sat in the doctor's office together. The nurse called Mom's name. We were led into an average-sized exam room. Dr. Kay sat facing Mom. He did the talking. He asked questions, directing them toward Mom. I remained silent until either Mom or Dr. Kay looked at me, expecting a response. Mom's story unfolded over about thirty minutes. After much discussion with Dr. Kay, in Mom's presence, he agreed to order the MRI. Thankfully, he was able to order it immediately.

Mom was anxious in the radiology department. I was allowed to talk to her while she went through the MRI machine. She was brave and didn't panic, allowing me to relax. When the radiologist provided the preliminary results, stating the test showed no abnormalities, I noticed Mom's eyes, a mix of confusion and worry. I knew this result was not a good sign because it meant that Mom's memory loss was *not* caused by a diagnosis that could be managed or cured. I already knew this. Really. Tears welled in my eyes. After more than six years of observing the symptoms and dealing with her excruciatingly slow decline, what did I think the findings would be?

We went back to Dr. Kay's office. After he reviewed the preliminary MRI report and assimilated all his findings, he confirmed a diagnosis of Alzheimer's. He was unable to offer any experimental medications to slow the symptoms or progress of the disease, stating that Mom's condition was too advanced for any clinical trials.

However, Dr. Kay started Mom on increasing doses of Trazodone, an antidepressant, hoping it would decrease her anxiety and allow her to sleep. If the medication was effective, after one month, he planned to add Risperidone (Risperdal), an antipsychotic medication that was often used to decrease delusions and paranoia.

Today, after over three decades of drug trials, the medical research has not proven successful in either curing or definitively arresting the progression of Alzheimer's. However, certain medications approved for mild to moderate Alzheimer's can temporarily improve cognitive function. These drugs include Aricept (approved 1996), Excelon (2000), Razadyn (2001), and Memantine (2003).

It wasn't until 2023 that the FDA approved Leqembi (lecanemab) for early-stage disease. It is an expensive infusion, but because it has been approved by the FDA, Medicare may cover it in certain situations. This medication has shown promise in slowing disease development by reducing clumps of amyloid-beta proteins in the brain for a limited period. However, the results are mixed regarding the benefits and efficacy of this medication. Another drug, Kisunla (donanemab), which may slow the progression of the disease in the early stages, was approved in 2024.

*****

Lori felt an urgency to get Rodney out of her life and Mom's, which was understandable. She had also suggested a few months earlier that I was in denial about the severity of Mom's disease. Her comment caught my attention and prompted me to evaluate my feelings.

I was quite familiar with denial—the first of the five stages of grief. Intellectually, I understood the process, having studied it extensively while working with oncology patients in my first job as an RN at the University. I had watched and counseled patients and their families as they navigated these emotions. The stages, as identified by the late Elisabeth Kubler-Ross, M.D., are denial (and isolation), anger, bargaining, depression, and acceptance.

For up to a year following a patient's death, I would check in with their families through telephone calls or visits. Through them, I witnessed firsthand how unique the grieving process is to each individual. I saw people get stuck in one stage or regress to an earlier one. Grieving is not a linear process; people move back and forth between the stages.

I considered that I might be stuck in the denial or bargaining phases myself. Over the previous few years, I had experienced periods of anger and depression about Mom's condition, but never total acceptance. In reality, I was quite aware of Mom's decline because I was so involved in her care. Yet, it was still so easy to slip back into denial or bargaining when she had a good day.

Ironically, here I was back on the grounds of the University of Minnesota Medical Center campus—memories of my cancer patients vividly coming to the surface as we left the hospital and walked toward the car. We held hands, walking slowly. As we approached the car in the parking lot, Mom stopped suddenly, turned, looked me in the eyes, and cried out:

"Promise me!" Her eyes bore into mine.

"Promise me, Kathi, that you will *never, ever,* put me in a nursing home."

My heart broke. A wave of despair surged over me.

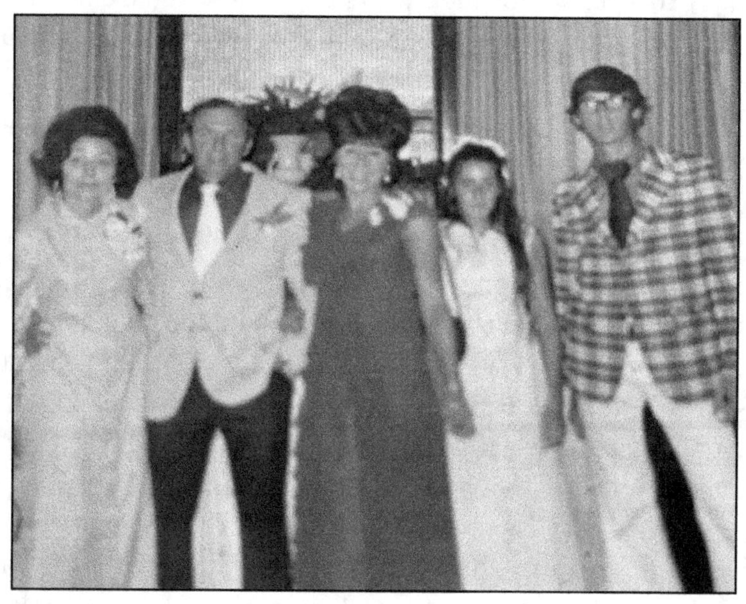

Aunt Gussie, Dad, Mom, Lori, and Dan

21

Relatives Reject Reality

After Mom's visit to the neurologist, events unraveled rapidly. Rodney and I sat down in the living room the day after Mom's appointment. She was in the bathroom trying to focus on applying her makeup. I did not let on that I was aware of his inappropriate advances with Lori, or that I had read his love letters. We were at a crossroads. We still needed Rodney to work with us.

"Rodney," I began, "we know Mom is getting more forgetful, and we know this must be getting difficult for you. How are you managing with her at home?"

He paused and said, "Sometimes it's frustrating because she doesn't remember how to do normal everyday things. I have to help give her a bath. But sometimes her aide, Candy, helps." He was silent for a moment. "She can't make coffee anymore, and I have to clean the house. She used to help with the cleaning. We would do it together." He paused. "But I can handle it."

He was clutching his coffee cup, looking down.

"Rodney, she is getting worse, and I worry about you," I said more softly. "Caregiving takes a real toll. You've done so much for her this past year. But every time I visit, I see more and more decline. She roams around the house at night. Her paranoia seems worse, and the delusions are more frequent, causing her so much anxiety. It took me almost two hours to help her with a bath today." I paused. "How're you really managing?"

"Well, it's hard," he replied. He fell silent.

"I know it is. I'm so sorry." I paused, allowing myself to feel my sadness. "Lori may have mentioned we're looking at adult foster homes for Mom. She needs specialized care and treatment. What did Lori tell you?"

"Yes, Lori did say something about that."

"Do you remember our conversation when you moved in? We talked about Mom's illness and the progression of Alzheimer's disease. We talked about how we would need to find a place for her when her condition required specialized care. We think it may be time. What do you think?"

"Yes, I suppose so. But if I quit my job, I think I could manage. I love your mother and will do whatever I can to help."

"Thank you, Rodney. We think it's time. I see your struggles with her and how frustrating it is for you sometimes. It must be difficult. Even if you are here full-time, her needs will stay the same. She requires daily monitoring, especially with the new sleep medication. Will you remind her to take her pill at night? We really do appreciate your help."

"Yes, of course I will."

"We are grateful for all you've done for Mom. Thank you for helping her stay at home for this long."

"Yes, just let me know what I can do."

"I will, Rodney. Thanks."

I had to maintain a good relationship with him and possibly run interference for Lori until we found a safe place with professional help for Mom.

*****

A few days later, I called Uncle Bill, my mom's oldest brother. He had not been privy to Mom's gradual decline in health over the years. We shared a special relationship that had been built on years of correspondence. He lived in Davenport, Iowa, about a six-hour drive from the Twin Cities. When I was growing up, he lived in Chicago and routinely wrote me letters and postcards. I always responded in kind, and he often told me how much he delighted in opening the mailbox to see a letter in my handwriting. Mom encouraged my relationship with him, happy that we were close; I believed she thought he was lonely because he was single.

When I was a sophomore in high school, Uncle Bill paid for me to fly to Chicago for the weekend, and he put me on a train back home to St. Paul. At that time, I had never been on either an airplane or a train. It was a special trip with fond memories of walking along Lake Michigan, visiting the Chicago History Museum, and eating at the revolving restaurant atop the Lake Shore Holiday Inn. Mom was waiting to hear the stories of my adventures when I arrived home.

In the summer of 1976, when I returned to Minnesota from my travels in Europe, I went down to Iowa to visit Uncle Bill. I sought his advice for ideas on how I might help Mom because I knew she respected him. As a child, I would hear them talking on the telephone and was aware that Mom often called him for advice.

That July, Uncle Bill listened quietly to my concerns about Mom. I told him about my friends who were passing through St. Paul on their way west. I shared that they had invited me to join them, but I was reluctant to leave Mom. I asked if he would give me advice on how to help her? He sat quietly for a minute, then he spoke gently, but firmly. He said he knew I loved my mother, but I couldn't change her situation—she had to initiate the change. He encouraged me to go to California that year.

Now, after asking for his advice about placement and strategic planning for Mom, hoping for compassion and understanding, my expectations plummeted.

He sounded agitated when he spoke. "I don't want to see your mother go into an institution. I would rather she die in a fire in her own home than be admitted to a nursing home! I spoke with her last week and she sounded just fine!" He was shouting, then stopped himself and quieted.

I had to regroup. My mind reeled from his distant and punishing attitude. He resisted the reality of what I shared about Mom's current condition. Finally, I opened up about how I felt: "I'm feeling overwhelmed and need your help because I'm finding it hard to manage everything." I paused a moment, but he was silent. "Please,

Uncle Bill," I pleaded, "would you come to St. Paul and stay with Mom for several days? It would give you a much better idea of her condition, and we could really use your support. I am so worried about her."

"No! I will not come. And I will not help you look for places to put your mother. She needs to stay in her own home!"

After processing our call, I called my Uncle Alex, Mom's brother six years her senior, and his wife, my Aunt Gloria. Their responses were not encouraging. They hadn't seen Mom for several years and did not realize how poorly she was coping at home. Both were on the phone and said, "There must be other options for Adele. She called us last week, and we spoke with her; Rodney was also on the phone. They seemed fine."

My aunt and uncle had busy lives in Wichita, Kansas, and didn't get to St. Paul often, so it was difficult for them to fully comprehend her situation. Mom spoke to them frequently and respected and loved them, as did I, but they offered no suggestions.

My mom was close to her siblings and their large families. We spent many happy times with them over the years. Throughout my life, Uncle Alex shared stories of his world travels, always with a twinkle in his deep brown eyes. Sometimes I didn't know if he was embellishing the truth because his stories were so compelling and his experiences extraordinary. Mom loved to be present when he shared his adventures, even if she had heard them many times.

When my uncles came to visit, my mother and her sisters, all of whom lived in St. Paul, coordinated gatherings. Gussie, the oldest of the siblings, had ten children; the youngest five were close in age with four of my siblings and me. When we were together, we delighted in talking, laughing, singing, and playing.

On Christmas Eve, we all crowded into Aunt Gussie's living room, circling the piano to sing celebrated holiday songs, including my favorites, "Silent Night" and "O Little Town of Bethlehem." Both Aunt Gussie and Mom had converted to Catholicism when they married, and Aunt Gussie and my Uncle Judd celebrated the sacred holiday in earnest. Santa Claus was a welcome guest every year during the evening festivities.

My parents always hosted the Fourth of July barbecue in our backyard, complete with firecrackers and sparklers for the kids. My dad did the grilling, and my mom made the salads and cut up watermelon. Even today, my cousins tell me what special memories they have of those backyard holiday celebrations "at Aunt Dale and Uncle Ray's home."

I loved and adored my vivacious Aunt Gussie and felt blessed that she was also my godmother. She wrote a children's book titled *Happy Days with Jackie,* which was published when I was a child. I received the book as a precious gift from her and remember Mom reading the stories to me. Today, a pristine copy of the book sits on display in my home office.

Surely, I thought, my aunt would come to our assistance. After all, she had seen Mom on several occasions in recent years. Many times, when I was in Minnesota, I would take my mom and Gussie out to lunch or dinner. With Mom's decline, those outings became less frequent.

I called my aunt to explain the situation—we were in a crisis, a turning point with Steve in the hospital and Mom's condition worsening. I told her about Rodney and his advances to Lori and related our concern about Mom staying alone with him for much longer. I said we were looking at alternative living arrangements for her. I confided that Mom's current situation with Rodney had been in place for well over a year, but with her decline, he seemed to have his own delusions about a romantic relationship with Lori.

Gussie, in her early 70s, was widowed and lived alone. "Men will be men," she said over the phone when I described the situation with Lori and Rodney.

"I'm sorry," I said questioningly. "Did you say 'men will be men'? What do you mean by that?" I was perplexed. She was silent for a few moments before she spoke again.

"Kathleen, I don't share your concerns. I've seen your mom and Rodney together, and they seem very happy," Gussie said, her voice turning sharp. "If he is willing to stay at the house with her, she should continue to live in her own home."

I had never had a disagreement with my aunt and was stunned by her comments. She didn't seem to think that Rodney's behavior was destructive. *What the heck!* Much later, as I reflected on her comments, I wondered if her attitude was just consistent with her generation's views.

I tried to communicate to her that the issue with Rodney was not the only concern. Mom's condition was rapidly deteriorating; she was no longer safe at home, and we could no longer rely on Rodney.

"Aunt Gussie," I said, "Mom cannot bathe or shower herself. She can't be left alone in the bathtub. Even getting her into a car is a major effort, as it requires many prompts. She still smokes and turns on the gas burner to light her cigarette." I waited for her to respond.

Like Uncle Bill, Uncle Alex, and Aunt Gloria, she said, "Isn't there something you can do to help her continue to live in her home? She seems fine when I call. In fact, Rodney and your mom called me the other day and said they are doing fine. They did say something about you and Lori taking your mom's money." She stopped and said nothing further, but her words hit me like a gut punch, deeply wounding my self-confidence and forcing me to doubt our plans.

Dismayed, I retorted, "That isn't true. I think you know that." I paused, but there was silence. "I'm so sorry you aren't willing to help us. Would you please think about the things I just shared?" More silence. "Good-bye, Aunt Gussie." I ended the conversation and hung up the phone.

Sitting with a cup of coffee and the hope of a prayer, I wrote a letter to Dad in my journal. I missed him terribly at that moment. He would know what to do. I wrote about the turmoil I was feeling regarding Mom and my heartbreak. I wrote: "How do I honor her dignity while ensuring she gets the care she needs?" Moisture filled my eyes as the tears flowed and the pages dampened. I set the pen aside and pushed my journal away.

I called Lori. After some contemplation and discussion, we concluded that our aunts and uncles did not know how to deal with the situation. They were in denial. Mom was their "little sister," the youngest. To recognize and accept her decline likely hit them hard and was a wake-up call to their own fragility. They were dealing with their own grief.

While my beloved Aunt Gussie lived into her nineties, with her mind largely intact, my Uncle Bill was diagnosed with late-onset Alzheimer's in his seventies. I often wondered if he experienced early signs and symptoms of the disease during the time we were trying to cope with my mom's decline, thus making the situation too distressing for him. Since he never married and lived alone, there was no way of knowing when his symptoms first became evident.

22

The Bully Boyfriend

Being unsuccessful in obtaining help from my aunts and uncles was heartbreaking. I hoped they just needed time to accept the truth about Mom.

Their rejection, especially Aunt Gussie's accusations about Mom's money, was painful. Deep down, though, I knew she was just trying to protect her sister, but she did not have all the facts. The reality was that Mom didn't have much money. She owned several certificates of deposit (CDs) with modest balances. She also received a fixed Social Security check. We would need to sell her house to pay for care.

We now knew Rodney and Mom had the attention of my aunts and uncles. Additionally, we discovered that Rodney had encouraged Mom to revoke the Durable Power of Attorney document that named Lori and me as her agents. On a visit to the bank, Lori was denied access to her account. The bank informed Lori that the document had been revoked; they confirmed that Mom and Rodney had been in the week before. The revocation meant that we had no legal standing to protect our mother or manage her financial affairs.

I imagined Lori's stress level was off the charts when she called me with this disturbing news. I was back in Seattle but had a three-day trip to Minnesota planned for the following week. The purpose of my visit was to continue researching potential places for my mom to live and to assist my sister-in-law in finding a suitable place for Steve. His physician confirmed he would be transitioning from a hospital rehabilitation program to a skilled nursing facility in the spring.

After Lori and I talked, I immediately called Mom. "Hi, Mom, how are you doing today?" Silence. "Mom, are you there?"

"Yes," she answered emphatically in an angry tone.

I started again, "Mom, Lori just called me from the bank. She was going to withdraw some money to bring over to the house so you have cash when you and Rodney go out. But Lori said she cannot access your accounts. Do you know why?"

"How dare you! How dare you and Lori steal from me!" Mom screamed into the phone; her agitation was palpable. I could almost feel her anger seethe through the phone line.

Stunned, I said, "Mom, Mom, I hope you know that isn't true." The force of her words hit me like a hard blow.

"Rodney told me what you've been doing." She was screaming at me. "He said you are putting me in a nursing home and that you are plotting to sell my house! I don't want to see you or Lori around here. How dare you? You stay away from us. Don't you ever come to this house again, ever!"

I tried to interject, but a feeling of hopelessness was coloring my already weary emotional state. Mom slammed the phone down. She clearly did not recall that Lori and I had discussed a possible move with her. In fact, she had visited the Hope House with us.

Distraught, I called Lori. After much discussion, I dialed our friend and lawyer, Ken, to assist us once again. I updated him on our most recent issue: we would now be facing a court hearing to obtain a formal guardianship or conservatorship for Mom. This court process, in which a judge appoints someone to make legal, financial, or healthcare decisions on behalf of a person deemed incompetent, is typically a last resort—a path I advised people to avoid, if possible. The process can be expensive, alienating, and difficult for family members. Every state has slightly different laws regarding the appointments, as well as the structure of these arrangements. Guardians typically handle personal needs while conservators manage financial matters. In some states, these duties may be combined.

Ken prepared me for what would be in store for us, and for Mom, if we pursued legal action. But, as I already knew, he admitted that without an appointment as durable power of attorney or agent for healthcare decisions, we had no control over Mom's safety, well-being, or her financial situation.

In competency disputes, courts often appoint a family member or relative as the guardian or conservator. In cases where disputes arise between adult children or other relatives, a judge may appoint a neutral party from a guardianship company to serve as conservator or guardian. While this stranger must act in the best interests of the protected person, this duty is limited by the fact that they usually do not know the individual personally.

While appointees from guardianship companies may do a great job, the family has little to no control over their loved one once a judge appoints a stranger. Some guardians and conservators work cooperatively with the family, while others do not. There have been, and continue to be, stories in the news about how some court-appointed conservators quickly spend down the accounts of the incompetent person; they neither solicit nor respect input from the adult children or relatives about what preferences would best serve their ward.

The most efficient way to manage an incapacitated loved one's wishes is to execute power of attorney documents and advance directives well in advance of a need for them. I knew this, and we had planned ahead. We had the fully executed documents in place.

Unfortunately, our careful work and planning were upended when Rodney guided Mom to rescind these appointments and to rebuke her own children. Rodney was living in her home, where we were now unwelcome. Rodney and Lori were at odds due to his inappropriate advances toward her. Mom was declining faster than we had anticipated, and we were all worried about our brother Steve. We couldn't help but think that Rodney was preying on all of us during this vulnerable time.

23

Crisis Mode

Distressed by recent events involving Rodney, I met with Ken the first week in February. We were now forced to rely on the legal system to gain control of my mom's situation. I had spoken with him on the phone, but we needed to discuss filing a petition for Mom's conservatorship in more detail.

Deeply saddened by the lack of support from my relatives, and Rodney's bold moves, I pushed forward. There was no time to waste. Rodney was working to get control over Mom and to keep her at home despite the thorough assessment from Dr. Kay, the neurologist at the University of Minnesota.

In his report on January 25, 1995, Dr. Kay outlined Mom's Alzheimer's decline and her "delusional thinking, her apraxia, and other significant cognitive deficits."

Apraxia is a neurological condition caused by damage to the parts of the brain that regulate motor planning; it is common in Alzheimer's patients. Although muscle activity is normal, the brain cannot deliver correct movement instructions to the body.

I witnessed the increased difficulty Mom had in getting into a bathtub or a car as she struggled to remember how to bend and lift her legs. Sometimes, when eating, she raised her fork and then stopped for a moment—as if she didn't recall how to put the food in her mouth. And her stops and starts when walking also told the story of her brain not giving proper instructions to her body. She required frequent prompting and reminders.

Further, Dr. Kay wrote in his medical assessment that Mom's "current living situation is marginal given the major problem of the tension and issues between Lori and Rodney." (I had discussed the situation about Rodney with Dr. Kay away from Mom's presence when I was there.) He stated that he was "inclined to favor nursing home placement," or, in Mom's case, placement in the Hope House group home. Of course, I had gone over this with Rodney after the January visit. While he feigned cooperation, he secretly worked against us.

*****

In February 1995, Ken Rhodes filed a petition in court for conservatorship of Mom, requesting that the court consider Lori and me as co-conservators. During my meeting with Ken, he advised me that the court would appoint an attorney to represent Mom. That attorney, he said, would likely listen intently to Rodney and my aunt.

Additionally, Ken stated that since Mom was able to walk, albeit laboriously, the judge would likely require her to be present at the hearing. This news was deeply disturbing. I was more familiar with judges appointing conservators based on a review of medical record documentation from physicians and other qualified healthcare professionals, along with interviews with close family members or friends. Not only was this troubling news, but the entire process would be expensive and draining of Mom's modest resources.

My heart ached at the thought of Mom standing in front of a judge, with others watching and waiting for her answers. Depending on her cognitive state that day, she might be confused, embarrassed, or simply frightened.

We discussed the potential outcomes with Ken. Lori and I agreed that we wanted to place Mom in the Hope House if we prevailed as conservators. Ken advised us that there was a possibility that the court would appoint a stranger as conservator. Further, if Rodney and my Aunt Gussie convinced Mom's attorney that they could keep her safe in her own home, the appointed conservator could opt to leave Mom in her house with Rodney.

I was overwhelmed with worry and cried myself to sleep every night at Lori's house. The thought of moving Mom out of her home was fast becoming a reality.

Once back in Seattle, Ken let me know that Mom's court-appointed attorney, Ms. Dee, would be calling to interview me. As a reasonable person who loved my mom and only wanted the best and safest placement for her, and as an attorney working in the long-term care profession, I assumed that I would find common ground and shared compassion with Ms. Dee.

Promptly at the scheduled time, I answered my phone to a cool, detached voice. "Hi, Ms. Hessler, this is Ms. Dee. I represent your mother in the conservatorship hearing. I have a few questions for you. This will be quick." I could hear the swishing of paperwork in the background. She started with quick, short questions that she should have already known the answers to. As we talked, Ms. Dee was all business, typing on the computer and appearing to have already decided what to believe. While I felt she discounted the history I provided by interrupting me several times, I considered that her fast-paced approach might be due to a heavy caseload or her sense of duty to carefully question family narratives to protect her client. Yet, she didn't inquire about how my mom was managing at home, or what my experience was in staying at the house with Mom and Rodney.

Then, adding to my frustration, Ms. Dee informed me that she was going to schedule another medical appointment for Mom. I asked that she first obtain Mom's medical records before taking her to another doctor. I provided the names of all the physicians and healthcare professionals my mom had seen, and mentioned that she could obtain the records from the doctors or directly from Ken Rhodes. She curtly ended the call, repeating that she would take my mom to see another physician, even though, weeks before, Mom had seen Dr. Kay at the University. I could not have been more wrong about finding common ground or compassion. I wondered why she called me.

Despite our conversation, on February 28, Ms. Dee took Mom to a new physician, who confirmed what her other doctors had been saying and documenting. This physician wrote: "As you know, this woman has significantly impaired intellectual and emotional functioning at this time and does need guardianship. I feel she can make elementary decisions with input from her family at this stage. She cannot care for her affairs in any complicated, complex, or detailed way."

Ms. Dee's decision raised a red flag because I knew she should have first reviewed all established medical records before subjecting my mom to unnecessary appointments or scrutiny. This was standard procedure, and she should have taken my background information and current observations seriously. I was incensed, but Ken said there was little we could do about her attitude, mentioning he had also tried to reason with her. He warned me again that Ms. Dee might find Rodney and Aunt Gussie's stories compelling.

Lori and I had both previously advised Ms. Dee about Rodney's inappropriate advances. As proof, Lori had saved the "love notes" Rodney had written and gave them to Ken so he could provide copies to Mom's legal counsel. Because Rodney had turned Mom against us, we were unable to visit her. Once Ms. Dee was appointed to represent Mom, we were definitively told to stay away from her until after the March 7 hearing—the day before my mom's sixtieth birthday. My heart was breaking piece by piece.

I flew back to Minnesota on March 4 and stayed with Lori. Meanwhile, Ms. Dee was actively interviewing and meeting with Gussie and Rodney. She also planned to speak to the staff at the Hope House, as she knew it would be the preferred placement if Lori and I were awarded the conservatorship.

After hearing our stories about Rodney and seeing the love letters he wrote to Lori, Ms. Dee requested that Gussie arrange a meeting with my mom at Gussie's house so that she could talk to Mom alone. The meeting was scheduled for two days prior to the hearing. I arrived in St. Paul the day before Mom was scheduled to be at Gussie's home for the appointment.

When Lori and I spoke to Ms. Dee about the "love letters," we asked her not to tell Mom about them because we believed it would be emotionally destructive for her to learn what Rodney had done.

However, Ms. Dee did not heed our recommendations. While at Gussie's home that afternoon, she read the letters out loud to Mom in the presence of Gussie. She explained to Mom what Rodney had done.

Just as Lori and I predicted, Mom became extremely agitated and angry. She started yelling that she wanted Rodney out of her house immediately. Mom was out of control, screaming. Gussie immediately called me on my work cell phone and asked me to come to her house. I was out doing errands and was able to get there quickly.

When I arrived, Mom was shouting, "Get him out of my house NOW! How dare he! I never want to see him again. How could he do this to me?"

Ms. Dee immediately started defending her actions. She told me that Mom had a right to know about Rodney's indiscretions. I was furious. I had no memory of ever seeing Mom so distraught. She turned to me, her face twisted in anger, tears streaming down her face, "Kathi, get him out of my house! Now!"

I went over to her and tried to put my arms around her. She softened a bit, but then pulled back and looked me in the eyes, "Kathi, can you help me?"

The problem was that Mom could not return to the house because Rodney was there. He had a lease, and we needed to give him a 30-day notice to vacate. However, neither Lori nor I could issue the notice, as we were no longer Mom's agents, or attorneys-in-fact.

Gussie said that Mom could stay at her house until after the hearing. Ms. Dee asked if I would go to Mom's home and get some of her clothing and medications so she could spend the next few days with Gussie. We had a plan. But I was beside myself, feeling a loss of control and sadness for Mom. I was furious with the attorney. But I wanted to cooperate to help Mom find calm. I was so worried about her.

I went to the house; thankfully, Rodney was not there. Ms. Dee had spoken to him and told him Mom would not be returning home, but that I would be coming by to pick up some clothes for her. Ms. Dee shared that she had informed him that she had disclosed his indiscretions to Mom. His response was bold; he said he was not moving out.

We were at the mercy of the court. If the judge appointed a stranger to manage the conservatorship, we might lose all say in Mom's care. While Aunt Gussie acknowledged Rodney's transgressions, she wasn't yet convinced that Mom needed to be placed in a group home or facility.

Fortunately, it didn't take long for my aunt's opinion to change. Late on the second day of Mom's stay, Gussie called me, distraught.

"Kathleen, your mother has been with me less than two days, and I'm exhausted." She paused for a moment. "She can't be left alone. It takes me over an hour to get her into the bathtub, and then I have to bathe her because she doesn't know how to use the washcloth!"

I thought I heard a deep sigh, but I remained silent.

"She can't do anything by herself," Gussie continued. "I can't even go outside and shovel my sidewalk. I'm so, so sorry that I didn't believe you. I agree—your mother can't live alone. She needs a full-time caregiver and a home that provides round-the-clock care. I'm so sorry."

While I felt a wave of relief that my aunt finally understood Mom's deteriorating condition, it was a bittersweet victory.

Mom was distraught and unconsolable. As people with Alzheimer's disease lose their short-term memory and cognitive functions, they may continue to experience lucid moments. More importantly, emotional memories are stored in parts of the brain distinct from those associated with recent memories. After she learned about Rodney's deceit, I talked with Mom daily. She was beside herself with grief. Her anger and pain were palpable and I wondered what lasting effect his betrayal would have on my mom's sense of safety? I wanted her pain to go away.

Separately, Gussie told Ms. Dee that she would no longer oppose Lori and me as co-conservators. She agreed with placement in a home, but not at the Hope House. She asked the attorney to consider recommending her sister be placed in a nursing facility that my aunt was familiar with and favored. Rather than checking out a new place without Mom, Ms. Dee took her to another strange place, putting Mom through more emotional strain.

*****

The hearing was held in the afternoon of March 7. Several of my siblings were present. Lori and I sat with Ken across the aisle from Mom, her attorney, and Gussie. My anger continued to simmer over Mom having to appear in person. The judge asked her to stand. The environment was strange and intimidating, and I could see that she was scared, slowly looking around, trying to understand what was happening. Rising timidly at Ms. Dee's prompt, she turned around as if looking to see where she was, bewildered. She was so anxious that she could not speak.

It was vividly clear that Mom did not understand the questions the judge had asked. I suspect she didn't understand why she was in court, much less remember anything her attorney had told her about the proceeding. At that moment, I believe the judge realized the severity of my mom's condition. He gently told her she could sit down. Ms. Dee stood and whispered into Mom's ear, prompting her to sit. This situation was a travesty, and I felt helpless.

In the end, the judge awarded co-conservatorship to Lori and me, which, in Minnesota, includes guardianship. Finally, a victory—although heartbreaking and at a huge emotional cost to my mom and our family.

24

Plans Unravel

When I left the courtroom, I felt like I was walking out of my three-day state law exams—relief, exhaustion, and the lingering fear of the unknown.

Mom looked sad and frightened as we walked out of the courthouse, then she started to cry. She was walking slowly while Gussie held her left hand. I went to her right side and wrapped my arm around her shoulder. She did not resist. Lori and my other siblings walked behind us. Mom did not react to seeing Sissy. Her projected anger was now appropriately directed at Rodney.

In the parking lot, Gussie repeated how sorry she was that she didn't believe us about the severity of Mom's decline. She said she knew Mom needed 24-hour care. For many years to come, Aunt Gussie would continue to apologize for not trusting us.

Mom's attorney left without speaking to either Lori or me. I thought, *Good riddance to you.* Even understanding her role as an advocate, I believe she put Mom through more heartache, strain, and expense than was necessary. Although confronting Mom with Rodney's letters may have ultimately helped our situation, I still maintain it was harsh and question whether it was necessary.

In any case, the hearing was over. The next day, March 8, was Mom's sixtieth birthday. Although fatigue had set in, we stopped for a bite to eat with Gussie. Then we took Mom back to my aunt's home. I hugged my mom long and hard, trying not to let her see me crying. She had to stay another night with Gussie because Rodney was still at the house.

Now that Lori and I were officially co-conservators, we could issue a 30-day notice for Rodney to vacate Mom's home. We asked Ken to issue the notice the next day on our behalf as conservators. Ken's plan was to go over to the house while I was on the plane to Seattle.

I was grateful that I had officially required Rodney to pay rent and sign a lease so we would not have to go through a formal eviction process—assuming he would leave after proper notice to vacate. However, it meant that Mom couldn't go back to her home. She had shouted over and over the previous few days that she never wanted to see Rodney again. The emotional trauma of Rodney's deceit held prominently in her mind.

The plan for Mom's birthday was for Lori and Sissy to pick her up at Gussie's home late in the morning and take her to lunch, where they would meet my brother Dan. Then, they would all head over to Hope House, where there was a room waiting for Mom. Dan and Lori's husband, John, had moved some of Mom's furniture and other things into the house earlier that week.

When Lori and I took Mom to Hope House weeks before, we discussed with her the possibility of living there. She said she would prefer to stay in her own home, but that it was a "nice" place. We told her Gussie would visit frequently, and Lori lived nearby.

I had taken substantial time off work in recent months and needed to get back to Seattle. My plan was to return in April, just a month later, to see how Mom was adjusting to her new place and to start dealing with packing up and cleaning her home. We would need to prepare it for sale so we could pay the monthly fee at Hope House. We didn't anticipate major issues getting her settled there.

I arrived back in Seattle still exhausted and filled with sorrow. I continued to find it challenging to accept that at sixty years old, Mom had progressive early-onset Alzheimer's disease and needed round-the-clock care. It felt like a bad dream that I was trying to wake up from, only to dream it again and again.

As I unpacked at home, my phone rang. I picked it up and immediately heard Lori's frantic voice.

"Kath, it was a terrible day! A terrible day! Mom is in the hospital for a couple of weeks. She broke down. It was awful—so, so sad! Poor Mom!" I heard Lori's muffled cries, interrupted by occasional sobs.

"Oh, Lori, I'm so sorry. Tell me what happened. Take your time." I held on, waiting for her to continue. Then, she related the scene earlier that day.

"Kath, Sissy, and I picked Mom up at Gussie's house about eleven this morning. She seemed genuinely happy to see both of us. We went to Embers, where Dan was waiting for us. We all had a good lunch. Mom ordered her favorite bacon, lettuce, and tomato sandwich. After we were done eating, the waitress brought a piece of chocolate cake with a candle on top. She lit the candle, and we all sang Happy Birthday to Mom. Mom was following the conversation during the meal and seemed to be enjoying lunch with us. She didn't talk about the hearing yesterday—as if it had been erased from her memory.

"Anyway, after we finished eating, I told Mom that we were going to Hope House. She didn't respond, so I didn't say anything else. When we arrived at the place, Sissy and I helped Mom out of the car. She seemed confused, but walked slowly with us up to the door, looking around at the big bare trees in the yard. We went inside."

Lori stopped and started crying again. "But Kath, once we got inside, I think she recognized the place from when you and I were there with her. She started yelling and screaming that she was not going to stay there. She became irate and turned to me—her face filled with fear. I felt horrible. She ran back to the door and exited into the front yard."

"Oh, Lori, I'm so sorry. Our poor mom." Tears welled in my eyes, but I didn't know what else to say. I waited.

She continued after a brief pause. "Dan was a few minutes behind us in his car. We all planned to meet at Hope House to stay with Mom for a while and help her adjust to her new surroundings. As he was parking in front of the house, he saw Sissy, me, and Mom inside the gated yard. Mom spotted him getting out of his car and took off running towards him. But he was on the other side of the tall black iron fence that surrounded the yard."

Lori cried again. "Mom said, 'Get me out of here! Danny, Danny, get me out of here!' "

Lori continued, "Mom screamed again and ran to the iron bars, grasping one in each hand as she yelled, 'Shit, get me out of here—NOW!' Mom looked at Dan through the openings of the black bars and continued to yell. It was terrible, Kath."

When Dan told me the story, he said he had never heard Mom utter a swear word in her life. He was shocked and devastated to see her pain. "I couldn't believe it," Dan recalled, his voice tinged with disbelief. "Mom just lost control, and it was frightening. She ran to the black iron gate, grabbed the bars, and tried to climb it. I'd never seen her like that." Even though it was years later when Dan related his memory to me over the phone, I could hear him crying softly, which caused me to tear up.

Once Dan saw Mom, he ran up to the gate and around onto the grounds to help her. Together, Lori, Sissy, and Dan guided Mom out of the yard and away from the home. They tried to calm her down, prompting her to position herself to get into Dan's car. Lori and Mom sat in the back. Sissy was upfront with Dan.

While all this was going on, the director at Hope House suggested Lori take Mom to Riverside Hospital Mental Health unit in Minneapolis, where they would treat her agitation. It was a short car ride over the bridge across the Mississippi River. Lori said that during the drive to the hospital, Mom continued to scream and yell, leaning over to pull at Danny's shirt, begging him to take her home.

25

Tulip Place

Isn't my new home pretty? Look at the bright yellow and red potted pansies out there in my garden," Mom smiled, pointing out the large bay window. It overlooked the main courtyard where several potted plants provided brightness to a gloomy spring day. She stopped for a moment and looked at me. "Isn't my new home nice?"

Mom was waiting for my answer. We had been meandering around the nursing facility's comfortable, clean surroundings, while I carefully watched her demeanor. "Yes, it is!" I replied. It had taken me a few seconds to respond; I was surprised at her lighthearted mood and willingness to acknowledge her new home. Mom—cute as ever in a pair of blue jeans and a stylish top—was walking with a steadier gait than I'd seen in many months.

Tulip Place was a private-pay skilled nursing facility in a quiet residential neighborhood in Roseville. Mom had been a resident in the home for a few weeks. She was admitted there instead of Hope House because the physicians at Riverside Hospital said her condition required advanced care.

She resided in Tulip Place's Memory Care unit. Her room was clean and spacious with a window looking out into a second courtyard, where a sprinkling of green buds were starting to appear on the trees. When I arrived, I went to her room, where I found her looking out the window. Her roommate, Cindy, was sitting in a comfortable reclining chair wearing one of Mom's sweatshirts—of which Mom was oblivious.

Mom spent more than two weeks at Riverside Hospital's Mental Health unit after her breakdown at Hope House on her sixtieth birthday. The physicians at Riverside treated her for anxiety, agitation, and delusions.

She had been through a lot during the past few months: Rodney betrayed her and was no longer in her life; her oldest son was in the hospital; and the hearing for conservatorship was confusing and humiliating. Moreover, devastatingly, we had moved her out of her home without her beloved dog and constant companion, Penny. Trying to move her to Hope House the day after the hearing had proved too much.

I knew from my research that too many changes for someone with Alzheimer's can be detrimental. In particular, a move to a different residence, or even a transfer to a new room in the same facility, can trigger trauma or a downward trajectory in a person suffering from dementia.

Surprisingly, the stay at Riverside Hospital provided Mom with some much-needed time and attention from trained professionals who were able to get her delusions under control—finally. The physician started her on a medication called Risperdal, which is used to treat certain mental mood disorders. It's an antipsychotic and can act as a mood stabilizer. (This was the medication that Dr. Kay planned to prescribe for her.) They adjusted the Trazodone she had been taking. They monitored and adjusted her medications to ensure she was at therapeutic levels before discharging her to Tulip Place.

Mom and I held hands as we continued on our self-guided tour of the facility, outside of the memory care unit. This was one of the many nursing homes I had visited over the past year, and was my top pick for her, but I hadn't envisioned her being admitted to this home so soon. After a few minutes, Mom stopped walking and turned to face me, waiting for me to turn to look at her.

"When can I go home? I miss my home. I miss my Penny. Who is taking care of my dog? Where is she?" Surprised, not expecting this twist in the conversation, I looked steadily into Mom's deep brown eyes. Tears were streaming down her face. I took a deep breath, trying to hold back my own muffled cry. I put my arms around her.

Mom had been at Tulip Place for a few weeks. I had called her nearly every day from Seattle before my trip here, and each time, she asked about Penny. Each time, I told her that Sissy had found a loving home for her dear little rat terrier.

"Mom, this is your new home now." I tried to take her back a few minutes. "It's a beautiful home. You're right. The garden is so colorful, and it's fun to watch the birds flit about in the aviary by the front door." I enunciated each word slowly and carefully, wishing I had the courage to respond directly to her questions about Penny, anxious to see if Mom would say more. "And your room is neat and pretty with the colorful comforter Lori bought you."

Mixed feelings of stress, guilt, and sorrow were like a knot in my soul. I felt miserable knowing Mom's independence was diminishing more rapidly than anticipated. My pain was a sharp ache that stayed with me day after day. I was angry that this disease was happening to Mom and affecting me and my siblings. At night—many nights—the tears flowed and dampened my pillow. My sleep was disrupted; I would wake up with my hands curled into fists, and a deep anxiety would come over me.

"Mom, I'm so sorry Penny can't live here with you. But Sissy found a good home for her." I hesitated.

"What do you mean she found a home for her?" Mom looked at me with confusion.

"Penny is living with a family in a residential neighborhood near Battle Creek Park."

"Oh, when did Penny go live with this family? Who is feeding her? I need to give them money if they are taking care of her." Mom's voice softened.

I looked at Mom and said, "The family that is taking care of Penny thinks she is so smart. Of course, we always knew she was a clever dog. They have two young children who love to play with her. They were looking to adopt a small rat terrier just like Penny!" I paused.

"Are you sure she is okay? When can I get her and take her home?"

"Mom, the family is taking good care of her. Sissy keeps in touch with them, and they take Penny on walks to the park every day. The kids, a boy and a girl, who are six and eight years old, will be out of school soon, so she will have even more attention."

"But I want to see her. I want to know she is okay. When can I see her? I need to see her." She raised her voice, but she didn't become belligerent, like in recent times. The medications really did stabilize her mood. While she was appropriately sad and grieving the loss of her dog, she was more herself than she had been in several years.

"Okay, Mom, I will find out if we can go see Penny," I said.

Mom was more active, walking faster than in prior months. Also, I was pleased to see that she had calmed down. She had more moments of clarity, although they quickly dissolved into confusion. Her delusions were gone, and her anger had subsided. Like a diabetic needs accurate insulin dosages to manage the disease and prevent complications, Mom needed these psychotropic medications to allow her a higher quality of life, free from agitation and delusions.

"Okay," Mom said as she turned and continued walking. "So, what do you think of my new home?"

"Show me more," I said.

*****

I arrived back in Minnesota in mid-April with plans to stay ten days, taking another short leave from work. The spring showers were sure to bring robust May flowers. I was ready for the spring bloom in more ways than one. I wanted a new beginning—a new season—for Mom and me, and our family. Certainly, the team of professionals here will provide her with the care and compassion she needs.

My plan was to become acquainted with Mom's new caregivers in the memory care unit and observe their interactions with Mom. I wanted to encourage her to participate in the activities offered, such as music or exercise classes, movie nights, crafts, or gardening. Also, I wanted the staff to get to know me, so when I called Tulip Place from my home in Seattle, they would know me as Adele's daughter and co-conservator.

In addition to daily visits to Tulip Place, I started sorting through Mom's belongings at home. Rodney was gone, and I was staying there now. The day after the conservatorship hearing, Ken had hand-delivered a 30-day notice to Rodney to vacate Mom's home. He had been paying rent directly to Lori on the first of the month. Although he had paid Lori for the month of February, the rent for March was not paid, as he had had no further contact with her after the revocation of our power of attorney.

A few days after Rodney received the written notice from Ken, my brother Dan and brother-in-law John went over to the house. They knocked. No response. They peered through the window of the kitchen door and saw Rodney standing in the dining room, looking at them. Dan spoke loudly, asking him to open the door so they could collect some of Mom's belongings. At first, Rodney hesitated, then he finally let them in.

An argument ensued when he opened the door. Then, Rodney grabbed a sharp, gold letter opener that Mom kept on a side table in the dining room. He pointed it at Dan. Dan and John pleaded with Rodney to put it down. They assured him they were just there to collect Mom's clothes and personal items. Rodney stood there, threatening to stab them if they came closer.

Dan picked up the phone in the kitchen and called the police, informing them that there was a man threatening him with a razor-sharp letter opener. Two police cars arrived within several minutes, driving up on the lawn close to the door—ready for anything that might transpire. Once inside, the police officers were apprised of the situation. The police listened to Rodney, too, took the letter opener from him, and suggested that he move out as soon as possible. He was gone the following weekend.

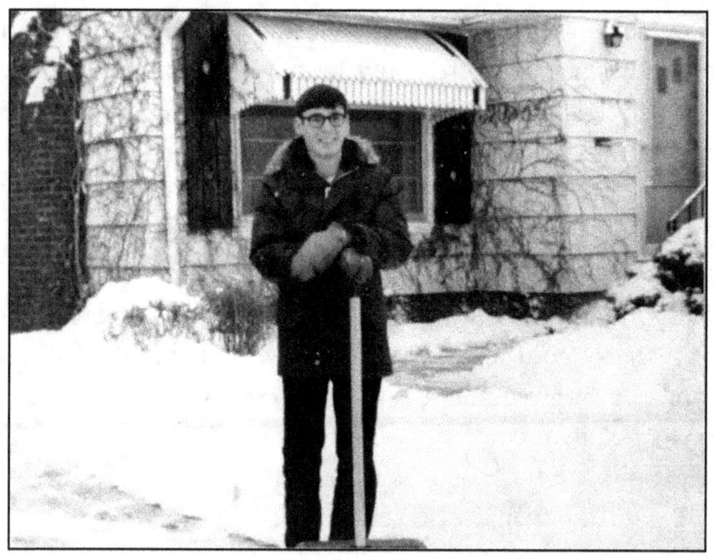

Dan shoveling snow at our family home

26

The End of an Era: 1963-1995

The house was quiet. Many years had passed since I was alone in our family home. As I reflected, I realized I had never spent much time by myself in our house on Norbert Lane. We moved there when I was seven; I left at eighteen. Now, returning as an adult, I felt lonely without all my siblings. While we had typical sibling arguments growing up, the current tensions among us were more serious, shaped by recent hardships.

We planned to put the house on the market in late May. Since it was now mid-April, it was time to sort through over thirty years of cherished belongings. I discussed my plans with Lori to stay at the house and start the sorting, but I shared that I wanted a few days alone to regroup. I didn't know what feelings would come back to me in the empty house without Mom there. I needed some alone time to grieve and to absorb whatever good memories could be recaptured.

My initial suggestion was to rent a storage unit and temporarily move Mom's belongings there. I favored waiting until Steve was out of the hospital to go through her possessions. I hoped that with time and healing on our side, we would be in a better frame of mind, and together, the process would bring us closure. It would have taken some effort to move the stuff and would have added an additional cost to Mom, so I understood the reluctance to do this. However, I believed it was a reasonable solution even though it didn't garner support from my siblings.

I had assumed, perhaps erroneously, that Lori, who often acted as intermediary among us siblings, would share my plans with everyone; this had been the case more often than not in our family. I relied on her communication. However, with Lori's busy life and all the events that transpired in recent months, I wasn't sure how much information had been communicated or whether my other siblings were aware of my plans. Given their work and kids' schedules, they were not always available when I returned to Minnesota, so I didn't always see them. Although Sissy didn't yet have children, she lived close to Steve's family and was helping his wife care for their children during his rehabilitation.

While I had anticipated that we would get together at least once during the ten days I was home to start sorting things out, it did not come to pass. This lack of coordination kept us from discussing or dividing Mom's things as a group. Many years later, my brother Dan told me he didn't know I'd been in town until after I was gone, highlighting the communication breakdown. Prior to my visit, Dan had made a list of the many items in the house and sent copies to everyone. In retrospect, I should have called him directly once I was home. Lori and Sissy knew I was in town because we talked several times.

Tensions ran high, and moving Mom to Tulip Place was a heartbreaking and unexpected change for all of us. We were each entrenched in our own grief, making communication difficult. I was exhausted.

We had worked reasonably well on Mom's behalf in recent years, but I often felt like an outsider. Lori, who took the lead on many things because she was local, sometimes disagreed with me. She would voice her concerns to my siblings, Sissy and Dan, rather than discuss them with me directly. They would sympathize with her, but they would not reach out to hear my perspective. Sometimes, it felt like two or three of them were a united front against me, unwilling to engage, only exacerbating misunderstandings.

With my background as a nurse and a lawyer, I am accustomed to figuring out problems and working toward solutions, even when conversations are difficult. But that approach did not always work well within my own family. It is easy to fall back into old childhood habits. In my family, this meant keeping silent and moving on instead of working things out. I found myself reverting to those patterns when around my siblings, not always seeking a resolution in a timely manner.

Many times, we were willing to move forward, never discussing the conflicts, the pain, or the harm. Apologies went unsaid, issues remained unresolved, and forgiveness unrealized. Sometimes anger and pain deepened, creating invisible walls. But after some time, we usually moved on, happy to see each other and acting as if nothing happened.

I didn't know if there was an issue this time or if there were real scheduling conflicts—but all these thoughts were circulating in my head. There was nothing I could do about my siblings' perceptions, or their own real-life concerns. And I had a busy schedule planned while in town. So, I buried myself in the work of clearing out the house. This was my only chance to go through things, since we had self-imposed deadlines to ready the house for sale.

Once again, Ken Rhodes was working with us and our realtor. Because I was behind in my work, I wasn't sure I could return for a closing in May or early June, if the house sold. I would do what I could, mindful that my siblings would have to carry a heavier load in distributing the household goods, selling or giving away what nobody wanted, and cleaning the house. In several preliminary conversations, we discussed how some household items should be distributed, specifically that any items given to Mom and Dad would be returned to the one who gifted them.

I went to a grocery store, retrieved six boxes, and labeled them— one for each of my siblings and me. As I sorted through drawers, closets, bags, and boxes of things, I placed childhood photos, school pictures, and projects that Mom had saved into the appropriate sibling box. Old memories surfaced, and tears streamed down my face.

We agreed that certain belongings of Mom's had memories for some, but not for others. We decided that if something was special to one and not the rest of us, that sibling should take possession of the item. I took several items and temporarily stored them at a friend's house in Minneapolis, marking them on the list Dan created. I suspected others might want a couple of the things I stored, but since no one was there to discuss it with me, I decided to hold on to them until I could talk with my siblings.

As time passed and events unfolded, we never discussed the items I secured at a friend's home. I now realize my actions created resentment. In retrospect, I wished someone had initiated a conversation with me back then, or that I had forced a discussion. Old habits.

I was not privy to how the rest of Mom's possessions were divided and settled among my siblings, except for a few items. Steve had always loved Dad's tall, wicker barstools downstairs in the recreation room, so his wife took possession of them. Mom often said that Dad bought the house because of the built-in bar in the "rec" room, which he duly decorated to look like a saloon. His purchase of a pool table was like the icing on the cake for a bar setting. We all learned to play. We spent many hours in that room playing pool or board games, watching TV, and entertaining guests. Mom's ability to shop and cook for many, along with her organizational skills, created an artful and festive atmosphere in our home during the days leading up to the celebrated occasions.

When I meandered upstairs to my childhood bedroom, memories flooded my mind. While growing up, my three sisters and I shared the upstairs, which was one large room with an adjoining attic and sloping ceilings on both sides. There were two cubbyhole storage places near the staircase that led down into the main living area. I loved the room's coziness with its wood paneling, built-in drawers, and a bookcase. It was my safe place.

Since Cheri and I were the oldest, we claimed the beds on the far side of the room, flanking the center window. My bed was on the right and hers on the left. The room was a place where I could go for quiet time to escape the chaos of our home. With the bedroom door closed at the bottom of the stairs, it was a great place of refuge. I loved to read, so I would either escape into a good book, write in my diary, or, when I was younger, play with my Barbie dolls.

I cherished my Barbie and her best friend, Midge. I also owned the handsome Ken figure, who came in his own mustard yellow Mattel storage suitcase. Another favorite, Barbie's little sister Skipper, was a birthday present from Mom and Dad. I had many of the original outfits and accessories for the dolls, including custom bedroom furniture, some of which my older sister Cheri loaned to me when she developed other interests, especially her love of music and the Beatles.

Mom knew how much playtime with the dolls meant to me. When I asked her if I could use the cubbyhole space for my Barbie's home, she emptied the blankets and sheets she had stored there. The main living area for my dolls was on the top shelf of the cubbyhole, and the bottom was their bedroom. Mom would come to see how I had arranged the furniture, praising my creative layout and offering some of her innovative interior design tips.

I had packed up my dolls and accessories, carefully labeling the boxes, when I left home after high school. I tucked them away in the attic. I had looked for them a few years earlier, trying to ease Mom's burden by taking my things. But I couldn't find them. It troubled me—these cherished belongings represented hours of fond memories. What happened to them? I wondered. I grieved them. How odd. Do people really grieve lost things? I always thought I would find them. I wondered if Cheri took them by mistake when she and her husband bought a house up north. But she said no—she only took her own childhood things when she settled. I inquired with my other sisters, Lori and Sissy, but no one remembered seeing any of my Barbie keepsakes.

Now that we had to empty Mom's house for good, I thought that by pulling boxes and bags out of the attic, I might find my possessions tucked into a far corner. There were more things stuffed into the attic than I realized. But my boxes were gone; my childhood treasures were likely lost forever. I paused for a few minutes to consider if I had taken them with me to Seattle. I had no such recollection. Rather, I recalled thinking that they were safer at Mom's house since I rented and moved frequently.

Surprised by my feelings of distress, I whispered: *They were just things. Just stuff.* I repeated this to myself as I wandered alone through the house, faced with so many memories. The heavy emotional loss spilled over into my sorting and packing. In my sadness and despair, I wasn't ready to let go. With the dolls gone, I realized they connected me to happy times in my childhood. Perhaps my focus on these 'things' was a way to avoid dealing with the slow, agonizing loss of my mom.

Most importantly, another realization dawned: I was upset about losing my Barbie and accessories because they reminded me of joyful times in play. Setting up a home for the dolls was my way of escaping Mom and Dad's fights, Dad's drinking, and sibling squabbles. They represented a sense of calm and a life that I did not have at the time. Once I realized I could still keep and cherish these childhood memories, I was able to begin to let go.

A couple of days of initial sorting passed. I moved around the house, taking mental inventory as remembrances peeked out from the different rooms. After wandering through the house and circling back several times, studying the amount of stuff to pack, dispose of, or sell, I felt overwhelmed. *What should I focus on?* I shed a few tears, had a glass of wine, and continued with my work. I knew my siblings and their spouses would continue what I started, so there was no real pressure, but I wanted to do my share.

My mom had boxes of unused stationery and an assortment of greeting cards. Some of the cards contained writing, but were incomplete, and some envelopes had partial addresses that demonstrated her intentions. I was troubled by the thought that she likely forgot what she was doing. She was always so thoughtful, and sent cards to people on their birthdays and special occasions.

Later, I discovered a box of note cards just like ones Mom had gifted me years earlier. They were blank inside, but the cover contained a verse by John Burroughs, an American writer. Born in the nineteenth century, he was known as a naturalist and nature essayist who was active in the United States conservation movement.

In addition to gifting me a box of the cards, Mom framed a copy of the note card's cover and gave it to me for Christmas one year. She said the verse reminded her of me, that it described me. I still have the framed card in my office.

The verse:

I still find
each day too short
for all the thoughts
I want to think,
all the walks
I want to take,
all the books
I want to read,
and all the friends
I want to see.
John Burroughs.

Mom understood me and wanted the best for me and for all her children. She did what she could to help us realize our gifts and to find our paths in life.

I left trails of tears in that house as I traveled back through time.

156

27

Forebodings

Preparing the house for sale was a daunting undertaking. I was just scratching the surface, quite literally. I spent several hours each day, and most evenings, organizing and discarding items. I cleared the attic, hauling out heavy black garbage bags filled with tax records and old bank statements from Dad's Texaco station business. I flipped through piles of paperwork, disposing of it or setting it aside for others to discard. I carried boxes of homemade Christmas decorations and strings of lights downstairs and placed them in the living room for my siblings to sort through.

When I moved to the kitchen on the morning of April 19, to start taking inventory and sorting through the cabinets, I turned on Mom's small portable TV. Before a picture came into focus, I heard the blaring words: "Breaking News."

I turned to face the small screen, learning that a bomb had gone off at the Alfred P. Murrah Federal Building in downtown Oklahoma City. It was later determined to be a powerful bomb ignited inside a rented Ryder truck by a U.S. citizen named Timothy McVeigh. In 1995, it was the worst act of terrorism in the nation's history, killing 168 people, 19 of them children.

The news was all-encompassing. I felt tragically alone standing in the kitchen listening to the broadcasts of the immediate aftermath. Already distressed by events in our family, I sank into a state of deep gloom and despair for all the families who lost relatives and friends that day. This tragic event highlighted my own fears about loss, reminding me of the fragility of life that my family was grappling with. What kind of world were we living in? There was no one to answer me.

Later that day, I took a break and visited Steve, who resided in the inpatient rehabilitation unit at Bethesda Hospital, located near downtown St. Paul. Fully awake from his coma, he was learning to walk again. He received intense physical, occupational, and speech therapy each day, but he was not recovering his short-term memory.

On occasion, my siblings and I used dark humor to lighten some of the pain. We joked, out of Steve's presence, that perhaps he had 'checked out,' so he wouldn't have to deal with placing Mom in a facility or cleaning and selling her house. I could visualize Dan looking through the boxes of stuff with my other siblings, unsure of what to do amidst the chaos. I could hear his jesting to my other siblings: "Steve must have seen this coming and decided to take a long vacation!"

In many ways, Steve was spared much of the emotional pain the rest of us endured. He never fully regained his short-term memory, but his long-term recollections of our family, as well as of Mom and Dad, remain intact. He loved our parents and still talks fondly of them every time we visit. He says he doesn't recall anything from that dreadful year of 1995.

After visiting with Steve, I went to see Mom at Tulip Place. I arrived at different times each day to introduce myself to the nurses and certified nursing assistants (CNAs) working the various shifts, and to observe the level of activity and care Mom received. It gave me the opportunity to meet the different caregivers and to put faces to names.

On the first day, I met and spoke briefly with Linda, the Director of Nursing (DON) for Tulip Place's Memory Care unit. She was a new hire. I had met the administrator during my tour of the home months earlier. I liked him okay, but he was mostly focused on business. He was polite enough, but not particularly warm. This facility was part of a large national nursing home company, similar to the one I was working for in Washington state. Tulip Place was a private-pay, state-licensed facility, but they chose not to apply for

Medicare certification, which prohibited them from receiving government funds. So, when Mom became eligible for Medicaid, we would have to move her.

The reason we chose this facility was the sixteen-bed, all-female memory care unit. Additionally, it appeared to be a clean and well-maintained facility. The first two weeks Mom was in Tulip Place, she was settled in a room on the main floor because the memory care unit was filled to capacity. While we waited for an available bed, Mom wore an ankle bracelet that set off an alarm if she attempted to exit, or elope, from the building. This safety measure is often used at facilities without a secure unit.

Over the previous year, I had been involved in my share of elopement cases. Whenever a client facility notified me that a resident had eloped, I would thoroughly investigate why and how the resident left the home undetected. This information allowed me to recommend corrective measures and defend the facility when necessary. While many residents were found quickly, sometimes, neither the resident nor the facility was so fortunate.

Coincidentally, the day I arrived back in St. Paul was the day a bed became available for Mom in memory care. Once she was settled in the unit, her ankle bracelet was removed. I was eager to help her adjust.

Each day I visited, I took Mom on a walk around the facility, inside and outside the memory care unit. We walked briskly, making the rounds of the rectangle-shaped building. One day, she outpaced me and walked ahead, as if on a mission. She darted into a small room to our left. As I got closer, I smelled the strong odor of cigarette smoke. It was the only smoking room in the facility. Mom detected it like a bird after its prey.

As I started to open the door, I almost ran into Mom, who came out smiling sheepishly like the little girl who had just eaten the last piece of chocolate. She had a cigarette in her hand, which I assumed was given to her by one of the smokers. I suggested she go back into the room and smoke it, and I would wait by the door. Mom had tried for many years to quit smoking, even experimenting with hypnosis, but nothing worked. *What difference did it make now?* I thought. Smoking was one of the few pleasures she had left.

*****

While in town, I scheduled a formal meeting with Linda, the Director of Nursing, to get to know her and to ensure she had the necessary information to meet Mom's needs. While explaining Mom's history and her recent stay at Riverside Hospital, I stressed that she was more stable than I had seen her in nearly three years. I asked Linda to open Mom's medical record to discuss her current medications. Linda sat with her arms folded across her chest, leaning back from the table. Her gaze occasionally drifted to her watch or the paperwork that lay on the table in front of her.

Because Mom's prescribed medications from a physician at Riverside Hospital included Risperdal, a psychotropic drug, the nursing facility was required to be vigilant in monitoring and assessing her continued need for it. Specific sections of both state and federal regulations governing nursing homes provide guidelines to facilities for monitoring residents who receive antipsychotic or psychotropic medications. Mom was also on Trazodone, an antidepressant. The regulations and guidelines are periodically updated, but the intent is to ensure that each resident's drug regimen is free from "unnecessary drugs." And all residents must be closely monitored for side effects of these medications.

When a resident exhibits excessive drowsiness, agitation, or lethargy from a psychotropic or antipsychotic medication, the physician must attempt a gradual dose reduction. Also, the regulations require gradual dose reduction attempts during two separate quarters within the first year of treatment, and annually thereafter. These attempts may be waived if the physician documents specific clinical reasons for maintaining the patient on the prescribed drug and established dosage.

Additionally, state and federal laws require licensed nursing facilities to hire a medical director—typically under contract—to perform administrative duties. These physicians also assess and monitor residents as needed. Facilities must ensure each resident is supervised by a physician and is seen at least every thirty days. At Oakwood, the medical director also served as Mom's physician.

Advising my clients heightened my awareness of the risks associated with prescribing and monitoring psychotropic medications. I had encountered nursing home medical directors who—sometimes at the request of a nurse—overreacted to the regulations by prematurely decreasing or abruptly discontinuing these drugs, even when they were effectively managing a resident's symptoms. These clinicians failed to recognize how these medications can significantly improve a patient's quality of life and overall daily functioning.

My mother was one of those patients.

As I sat with DON Linda, my spirit sank; her body language remained aloof and dismissive. Nonetheless, I shared my mother's history of paranoia, explaining that for several years, she believed my sister was stealing from her. I described her delusions, anger, agitation, and physical decline.

I detailed her experience at Hope House and the circumstances leading to her admission to Riverside Hospital, where she was prescribed Risperdal and Trazodone. I informed Linda that the hospital physician kept Mom there until her medications reached therapeutic levels.

Finally, I shared that I had witnessed substantial improvement in Mom's quality of life. She was calmer than she had been in three years—moving with more confidence and agility, free from agitation and delusions. I concluded by specifically asking Linda to discuss my mother's care with the facility's medical director—who was not available that day. I emphasized the importance that she remain on these medications.

Because my intuition was strong and I felt uncomfortable with Linda's lack of enthusiasm, I wrote a note and placed it on top of my mother's medical record to ensure the medical director and all the nurses would read it. As Mom's co-conservator, I insisted that they call me before making any changes in her medications, especially the psychotropic drugs. I hoped my note, taped firmly in place, would speak louder than I felt I could at that moment.

Later that week, before I left town, I had the opportunity to meet with the medical director. We had a brief conversation, which made me feel a little better, though he did not instill confidence.

28

Precious Penny

Where is my Penny? Why isn't she here? Why can't she live with me?" Mom repeated these questions every day that April when I visited her at Tulip Place.

"Where is my precious Penny? Why can't I see her?" Her inquiries echoed each visit. Her confusion was unremitting. At first, I thought these questions would pass. She did not remember that her dog was living with another family, despite my reminders. I was worried about her.

Penny had been Dad's dog. After he died, Mom grew increasingly attached to the small multicolored rat terrier; she was smart, obedient, and a good companion. Like two souls brought together by loss, Penny and Mom relied on each other after Dad passed.

Tears streaming down her face, my mom asked, "When can I go home? I miss my home. What am I doing here anyway? Where is Penny? Who is taking care of her?" She sobbed.

Unfortunately, I had not considered how being separated from her dog would affect Mom. So many things had occupied my mind that spring: Mom's breakdown; her move from home, to hospital, to facility; and preparing her house for sale.

Losing a pet is devastating for anyone. Despite dementia and memory loss, emotional attachments persist. Mom's connection to Penny prevented her from forgetting her beloved pet. People with dementia mourn, and Mom was clearly grieving. Uncertain how to help, I thought taking her to see Penny might ease her sorrow. Earlier in the week, I had taken Mom out for lunch at a nearby restaurant. It was slow; I had to remind her to lift her feet to get in and out of the car, and prompt her to eat. Still, she tolerated being out for several hours.

I had consulted with Sissy and Lori about taking Mom to visit Penny, sharing my thoughts about her mourning the loss of her dog. I asked if either of them could take her to see Penny in the next week or two. I was returning to Seattle in a couple of days, and I didn't think I would have time. Lori was clearly overwhelmed by her young children, work, and preparations to sell the house. She said she didn't have time to take Mom, which I understood. Sissy was skeptical that this would be of any help. I felt the same uncertainty, but the enduring sadness in Mom's voice made me realize I had to try.

That day, as the sorrow in her voice returned with renewed intensity, I felt my own emotions shift from uncertainty to determination. Her constant questions about her sweet dog tore at my heart, stirring an urgent need in me to help. By the end of that visit, my sense of responsibility outweighed all hesitation. I would find a way to take her to see Penny before returning to Seattle.

Sissy gave me the new owner's phone number. When she contacted the Dodds about taking Penny several months earlier, she had explained Mom's situation. So, when I called Mary Dodd, she was happy to coordinate a visit. She said they lived two blocks from Battle Creek Park in St. Paul, and we could take Penny for a walk there.

When I saw Mom the next morning, I asked her if she would like to go with me to see Penny.

"Oh, yes! Kathi, can we really go?" She smiled and reached out to hug me.

"Yes, Mom," I said. "I called Penny's new owner yesterday, and she said we could come today if you want to see her."

That cool, crisp Saturday in late April was sunny and dry. I pulled up in front of their house, in a neighborhood much like the one from my childhood. The young couple and their children welcomed us warmly into their cozy, clean home. Mom's tension and bewildered expression melted quickly when Penny darted into the room and ran directly to her. A smile slowly widened across her face, then grew bright as she recognized her cherished pet—her momentary happiness a bittersweet moment for me.

Mom and I walked slowly to the park while I guided Penny on a leash. The fresh air lifted my spirit. Spring greeted us with the sweet smell of lilacs, and the sparse green buds on the oak trees lining the park paths gave me hope for new beginnings.

Penny was well-behaved—almost as if she were begging, 'Please take me home to be with my mom.' During our walk on the trails, her tail was wagging furiously as Mom bent down several times to hug and pet her.

As we approached the house on our return, I said, "Mom, I think Penny likes her new home; it's so close to the park. Her new owners are very nice. And their children seem to have lots of energy to play with Penny. What do you think?"

"Yes, I agree," she said. "I miss her, but I think she is happy. Are you sure, though, that she can't live with me in my new home?" Her sadness tugged at my heart like the leash I held tightly. I watched Mom's mournful face as she again bent down and petted Penny with gentle hands, mirroring my inner struggle between hope and helplessness.

My heart was aching for my mother, who, at sixty years old, had to leave her home and her precious pet. Although some of her long-term memory was still intact, the disease was robbing her of so much. I tried to pull myself together as we knocked on the door of the Dodd's home again. Mary, her husband, and their children were waiting for us. They invited us back into the house for a short visit.

"Thank you for letting us see Penny and take her for a walk. It means so much to us," I said gratefully.

"Yes, thank you," Mom said. She continued in her soft voice, "Did I pay you to take care of my dog? I must give you some money since you are feeding my Penny." Mom looked at me and whispered, "Do you have money to give them?"

"Oh no, but thank you," Mary interrupted. "We have enough food to take care of Penny. And as you can see," she said as she waved her hand over the pet toys on the floor, "Penny has lots of toys too. We love her. Noah and Lily have fun playing with her." The children were nodding as Penny let them pet her. "We take her on walks every day. I know she misses you, Adele, but we are trying to help her adjust. Thank you for trusting us with her."

Mom looked into the eyes of the sincere and kind woman. "I miss her too. Thank you for loving her," she said quietly and turned to the door. I couldn't tell if she was starting to cry. Mom was quiet when we got back into the car. The weight of the visit sat between us, her silence heavy with emotion.

As I drove, reflecting on our visit, I spotted a Dairy Queen. Seeking comfort for both of us, I pulled into the parking lot. I asked Mom if she would like an ice cream cone, or a Dilly Bar—one of her favorite treats at the DQ.

When we returned to the facility, we sat together in the lounge before I gave her a long hug goodbye. That day, Mom didn't mention her precious Penny again.

In the following weeks, she asked about her, but less often. Each time, I would answer, "Mom, when I was in St. Paul, we visited Penny in her new home. We took her for a walk in the park, and I could tell by the way she stayed close to you that she misses you, just like you miss her. But she also seemed happy living with children who take her for walks every day."

"Oh, yes. I remember," she would say. I don't know if she did, but she seemed to experience more peace about her dog—or so I wanted to believe.

29

Long-Distance Caregiving

I returned to Seattle the day after I took Mom to see Penny, but I felt unsettled. The need to stay connected to the nursing facility personnel and to my family occupied my mind. Our conversations about Mom's needs and her struggle to adjust to the memory care unit weighed heavily on my heart. This experience underscored the complex emotional and logistical challenges inherent in long-distance caregiving, especially during periods of transition.

I called the facility every few days and asked the staff to put Mom on the phone. She always seemed happy to hear my voice. When she had lucid moments, the calls were pleasant, even though they digressed into confusion. In addition to the phone calls, I mailed her short notes and postcards to brighten her day.

During my phone calls with Mom, I focused on good memories—walking, biking, baking, and shopping together. I told her I'd always admired her fashion sense and how fun it was to have her help me pick out a new dress for Easter or a school dance, followed by lunch—just the two of us. Sometimes she remembered the stories; sometimes she did not. Sharing them gave me comfort, and occasionally, they triggered her recall. It wasn't clear how long those memories would continue to stir within her. One day, I shared a story about the time I didn't make the volleyball team in eighth grade. Softly, over the telephone lines, I heard her say, "Yes, Kathi, I remember that; you cried."

Mom had always been astute at making me feel better when I had bad days at school, performed poorly on a test, or wasn't chosen for a school play or a sports team. She would tell me that other opportunities would come along, and not to let a setback stop me from trying out for the next activity. She was so right. Her message of picking yourself up and moving on was always accomplished with empathy and compassion.

As her memory faded and it became harder to talk on the phone, I grew increasingly frustrated with the distance between us. At that time, there were no Zoom or FaceTime technologies to facilitate communications.

In addition to my personal struggles, I was dismayed when I listened to some of my client nursing home administrators' opinions that adult children of nursing home residents who live out of town are often considered "out of sight, out of mind, and out of touch." I guess this wasn't much different from how some families view siblings who live out of town. In many cases, this might be accurate. In my case, it was not.

These perspectives made it clear to me that staying involved as a long-distance caregiver takes real effort. In some ways, it may even be harder than for some family members who live nearby. Sometimes, people view the long-distance caregiver as an interloper and do not give them the opportunity to participate in the care. Even with today's technology, maintaining active involvement still requires concerted effort.

Aware of these biases, I took extra steps to inform DON Linda that I intended to stay actively involved in Mom's care even though I lived in Seattle. I told her that as a co-conservator with Lori, the facility should contact both of us for urgent or emergent matters, or if there was a change in Mom's condition or medications. I was shocked when she said their only obligation was to contact one of us. I insisted that she understand she was obligated to inform both of us, as court-appointed co-conservators.

Although Mom lived in the nursing home in the days before Skype or Microsoft Teams, telephone conference calls were possible in the mid-1990s. While facilities had the capability to set up such calls for the requisite quarterly care plan meetings, many begrudged doing it, as I had experienced.

Under state licensing laws and Medicare nursing home regulations, facilities are required to schedule a care plan conference every three months and whenever there is a significant change in a resident's physical or mental health between quarters. The facility is required to invite the resident if the resident is able to attend and understand the purpose of the meeting. The home must also send a notice (an invitation to attend) to a resident's guardian, conservator, power of attorney, or designated family members involved in the care.

Initially, the staff resisted my request to set up a long-distance telephone conference call so I could attend the meeting. They stated that they did not have the capability to set up such a call, and because Lori would be present, I did not need to be. However, I knew better because my clients routinely discussed the telephone care plan conferences they set up for out-of-town family members. I persisted in my request to be included. Finally, one of the nurses agreed to organize the calls so I could participate. Lori would inform our other siblings so they could decide whether to attend.

*****

The Centers for Medicare and Medicaid Services periodically updates the voluminous nursing facility regulations. In 1993, when I first began working as an attorney in the long-term care profession, I was informed that nursing homes were subject to more regulations than any other industry in the U.S., except for nuclear power. I am not certain whether this was accurate or still true today, but I had read the extensive regulations at night and on weekends during my first months on the job. They were my guide in providing proper legal advice to my clients and in advocating for Mom.

Medicare nursing facility regulations were developed in response to the federal nursing home reform legislation passed by Congress in 1987. Historically, the public believed that many nursing home residents were medicated for the convenience of the staff. The Reform Act and subsequent regulations, which overhauled the industry, aimed to change the way nursing homes were operated, ensure the safety of all residents in a home-like environment, and set quality care standards, medication guidance, and staffing requirements.

*****

One day, while at work in Seattle, I received a call from DON Linda. She was talking loudly and fast, obviously upset.

"Hello, Kathleen, we just medicated your mother with Haldol. She was belligerent. She grabbed my dress at my chest and shoved me up against the wall, demanding that I take "her" dress off. She accused me of stealing her dress!"

"What?" I was stunned, not quite registering what I was hearing. "I'm sorry, I don't understand. She has been doing so well since she's been on the Risperdal and Trazodone. She hasn't had any episodes of paranoia, delusions, or belligerent behaviors since admission to your facility." I waited. There was silence at the other end of the phone. "Has she had other episodes in the past days or weeks that I'm not aware of?" I demanded.

Linda responded slowly, hesitating as she spoke. "Well, our medical director took her off those medications a few days ago. The regulations require that we take residents off psychotropic medications as soon as possible."

I couldn't believe what I was hearing. When I was in St. Paul in April, several weeks earlier, I spent time with this nurse and the medical director explaining that my mother was doing so much better on these medications—better than she'd been doing in over three years. I talked to them. I informed them that I was aware of these regulations and understood the requirement for gradual dose reduction—unless clinically contraindicated. I stressed that my mom had only been on these medications for a couple of months, and they were making a significant difference in her quality of life. They witnessed her calm behavior and her alert, active state. They were privy to her medical history—*if* they had read the records provided by the mental health professionals from Riverside Hospital, who took weeks to prescribe and titrate the dosages to meet my mother's needs.

Anger seeped through me. I was momentarily at a loss for words, then I could not stop myself.

"What do you mean? I sat down with you and spent time sharing my mother's medical history and what she had been through. I told you the Risperdal was helping her function better than she'd been doing in several years. I requested that you call me before making any changes to her medications. This was your responsibility."

I continued my rant. "She was doing so well, and her delusions were under control. I'm her daughter and her legally appointed co-conservator. I provided you with the information necessary to care for her, and now, she may never regain the level of functioning she had just weeks ago." I didn't breathe before continuing.

"By ignoring her medical history, you erased every step forward she made in living a higher quality of life. Have your medical director call me—he needs to reinstate her prescribed medications immediately! I cannot believe you disregarded the treatment plans of expert mental health professionals."

I stopped. I wanted to say I wished my mother had slapped her hard and ripped her dress, not just grabbed her. I was beside myself with anger.

Later that day, the medical director called and agreed to restart my mom on Risperdal and Trazodone. Still, I knew it would take time for her to return to a similar level of functioning using the original dosing methods. When someone is suddenly taken off medications that need time to build up in the bloodstream and tissues, it's difficult to achieve the same results quickly. At a minimum, it would probably take several weeks.

I felt captive to the facility with these seemingly non-compassionate people. After the incident, I immediately called the administrator and discussed the issue, devising a plan to move forward. Several weeks later, in early July, I spent hours writing a four-page letter to him, copying Lori, the medical director, and DON Linda.

I needed to put this incident in writing to demonstrate the gravity of their actions. They had taken away what little autonomy and quality of life my mom had left. I needed to express loudly and clearly that I intended to stay involved in my mom's care and would continue to try to cooperate with them to achieve that end. I was tempted to call the Minnesota State Department of Health to file a complaint against the facility, but I thought Mom would be better off at this juncture if I tried to work with them and provide education on these serious issues.

In my letter dated July 6, 1995, to Mr. John Berger, Administrator, I wrote, in part:

Thank you for the time, attention, and prompt action you took on my concerns a few weeks ago when I called about my mother, Adele Hessler. Since we spoke, both Linda Smith and Janet Doe have called me to further discuss my concerns. We now have a plan of action in place that I hope will help promote communication between the Alzheimer's unit and me.

However, the experience of the past month was very traumatic for my mom and quite discouraging for me (especially since my brothers and sisters and I went to great pains and did ample research to find a facility we thought suitable for our mother). Due to the seriousness of this situation and the numerous concerns that have been raised, I feel compelled to express these in writing.

Despite my geographic distance, as the daughter and co-conservator of Adele Hessler, I have been very involved in my mother's care for the past several years.

I went on to provide the Administrator with a short review of my mother's past, the medications she was on when admitted to their memory care unit, what happened when the medical director abruptly discontinued these medications without notice to me, and a review of the regulations pertinent to this issue, concluding with my expectations going forward.

I advised the administrator that I had spoken with the medical director and asked him to contact the physician at Riverside Hospital who specialized in antipsychotic medications; I provided him with the physician's name and number. I wrote that I set up a weekly call with the memory care unit to receive updates about Mom. Finally, I confirmed my expectation of being included in all care conferences. In closing, I said:

I believe I am a reasonable person, given cooperation from other reasonable people. Long-distance caregiving may create some difficulties, but with a little effort, I believe it can be a positive experience for everyone; most importantly, I think it will serve my mother's best interests. I will be back in the Twin Cities for a few days in late July. I will stop in to see you. Again, thank you for your prompt attention to these matters.

When I visited again a few weeks later, Mom was not quite as active as she'd been; I could see she was readjusting to the medications, although she continued to experience delusions.

*****

I lived and breathed nursing home care from a work and personal perspective. I was a daughter, a co-conservator, a registered nurse, and a lawyer in the nursing-home industry. I wanted to be just a daughter when I visited my mom. I didn't want to be ever vigilant and have to monitor every aspect of her care. It took a lot of time and energy, but I knew it was necessary. I knew the industry, I knew the laws, and I was determined to make sure she received the best care. With that said, I made every effort to collaborate with the staff.

While it was difficult to watch others take care of my mom, I knew some residents thrive in memory care units where staff are trained to understand their needs. I was aware that there were good homes that did a wonderful job working with memory-impaired residents and where staff listened to and worked diligently with families; in the course of my work, I had visited many of them.

While I was extremely disappointed in Tulip Place, it wasn't practical to move Mom again. Lori and Sissy visited frequently, as did Dan and other family members. We had eyes and ears on-site, and I worked hard to coordinate calls with the staff.

Even weeks after restarting the medications, Mom did not enjoy the level of calm she had experienced in the previous months. The physician ordered Haldol and Ativan as one-time—as needed—doses, to be used only if the staff was unable to redirect or calm her during episodes of violence or distress. However, I made it clear to the facility that they were *not* to administer Haldol to my mom without calling me first. I informed them that regardless of the time—day or night—they were to call me and put Mom on the phone. Even back then, I kept my cell phone with me at all times.

One night, alone in my apartment in Seattle, I awoke to the sound of my phone ringing. A glance at my clock showed it was two in the morning. The first thought, in my sleepy haze, was that something had happened to Mom. I grabbed my phone, my hand unsteady, and answered the call.

Without the opportunity to say hello, I heard, "Is this Kathleen? I'm Kim, the nurse on duty tonight at Tulip Place." She was talking fast; I was still groggy, trying to register who was calling. "There is a note in the chart to call you. Your mother is very upset. She's been wandering the hallways for nearly an hour, and she just picked up a chair and threw it at the door. She is yelling and screaming. I need to give her some Haldol, but there is a note on her medication orders to call you first—before I administer it."

"Please put my mom on the phone right now," I said as I became more alert.

The nurse must have handed the phone to Mom because I heard her soft voice. "Hello?"

"Hi Mom, this is Kathi. How're you doing?"

"Oh, hi. So nice to hear your voice. How're you, Kathi?"

"I'm fine, Mom. Tell me about your day. I miss you." There was a moment of silence before she grasped my words.

"I'm okay. There are nice people here. I have a pretty room."

Mom and I chatted for a few minutes, and I could tell she was calming down. I must have dozed off for a minute, because the next thing I heard was the nurse's voice: "How did you do that? As soon as your mom started talking to you, she relaxed and calmed down. Immediately, I've never seen anything like it. She was so upset, and nothing we tried calmed her down."

"I know and love my mom. We have a special connection; sometimes she just needs to hear a familiar voice."

"Okay, great. I'll help her back to bed now. Thank you so much. Good night."

"Thanks for calling, and please call me anytime something like this happens." I hung up but was unable to fall back to sleep.

Lori and I collaborated the next day, brainstorming ways that might help Mom relax. Mom loved music, so we discussed bringing in CDs of her favorite artists. When she did, Lori asked the staff to play the familiar music when they put Mom down at night. We also suggested they play the music when she became agitated or disruptive. The difference in her demeanor when they turned on the sounds of the big band music, Frank Sinatra, or Johnny Cash tunes surprised the staff. When I visited, my heart warmed when I watched Mom sway to the music that she had enjoyed dancing to just a couple of years earlier. Her body relaxed, relieving tension.

Long-distance caregiving, while challenging, can be effective and rewarding. I felt more connected when I was involved in Mom's care. I may not have been as communicative with other family members as I could have been, but I spoke with Lori often. On occasion, I sent copies of letters to my siblings to keep them informed about Mom's care.

It is not uncommon for resentments to build among caregivers within the same family, especially when one person feels they are carrying a heavier load than others. Each caregiver has a unique perspective and special gifts. For example, Lori loved to make sure Mom had stylish, clean clothes and earrings to match, just as she knew Mom would want. She paid attention to Mom's dignity and other important daily matters. Sissy was flexible in her schedule and able to visit Mom at various times of the day or evening. Dan lived fairly close to the facility and was able to visit frequently at mealtime. Cheri and her husband visited Mom intermittently.

When everyone is dealing with their own family issues and other life stressors, there is no easy answer on how to communicate or collaborate effectively. I wasn't always aware of what others were doing for Mom, as they were not always informed of my involvement. Sharing and coordinating information requires effort, but it's imperative for success in long-distance caregiving.

30

A Bit of Calm

Mom was settling into Tulip Place. Mercifully, she did not know her house had been sold. We had funds for about two years in a private-pay home. At sixty, her body was relatively healthy due to regular exercise and a balanced diet—although she had smoked for many years and had a fondness for sweets. She walked slowly and with purpose around the unit, sometimes with a shuffle. She accused people of stealing from her. Although she resumed her antipsychotic medication, she never fully regained her previous level of functioning.

Lori and I knew we needed to complete the paperwork to qualify Mom for a Medicaid-certified facility before her funds ran out. But we wanted to place her in a certified facility before she qualified. Although some homes have a limited number of Medicaid beds, they usually plan ahead to ensure a bed is available when a private-pay resident's financial status changes to Medicaid. While private-pay residents are more profitable, federal law requires a certified home to accept a current resident's transition to Medicaid once they become eligible.

For the time being, despite issues with her medication, we kept Mom at Tulip Place, remaining vigilant about her care. I spoke weekly with the director of nursing and often with Mom's nurses, but I never warmed to them as I would to the staff at her next home. My mood lifted with the warm weather, and I took comfort knowing Mom could wander in and out of the unit's courtyard, enjoying the fresh air and garden.

By late summer, my siblings and I hoped for calm and stability in Mom's condition. Nearly two years into my job, I continued to learn more about the operations and legal issues associated with long-term care. Commuting one hour each way daily from Seattle to Tacoma made for long days. Adding the stress of dealing with Mom and Steve's health had left little time for a social life.

Yet, throughout this period, I stayed in close touch with my cherished group of friends from the hospital where I worked during law school. We met at Green Lake on weekends to run the three-mile loop and eat breakfast afterward. Sometimes, we entered ten-kilometer races sponsored by Seattle businesses. I drew the line at marathons—I didn't have the drive to train. My best was a half-marathon. Still, I cheered my friends on when they crossed the marathon finish lines.

These friends were special, and I treasured my time with them. Since they worked in healthcare, they provided invaluable advice and support as I coped with the lingering loss of Mom. It was an indefinite loss, a type of grief that does not allow for finality, like a death. The years of slow decline are filled with emotional turmoil because a person with Alzheimer's is physically present but often mentally absent. My siblings and I struggled to support each other, each navigating grief in different ways.

I was trying to recover from the past six months and found comfort in the company of other friends too. One night in late June that year, Jessica called; I hadn't heard from her in months. She was an attorney I met while working as a contract lawyer. She invited me to dinner with her brother and a friend who were in town. They picked me up on their way to a waterfront restaurant, which was near my apartment. Unbeknownst to me, Jessica had told her brother, Keith, and his friend, Tim, that they were picking up "Keith's date" for the night. Keith, a divorced father of two young children, lived in Boulder, Colorado, where he worked in research at a local university.

Keith and Tim were in town to climb Mount Rainier. I was interested and asked them a host of questions. Before law school, I hiked, climbed, and skied with the Seattle Mountaineers. Although I still loved these activities, I didn't have time for them. Still, I enjoyed hearing others' stories. I regularly attended Seattle Mountaineers' events, which sometimes featured mountaineering expeditions to Mount Everest. My interest in climbing, particularly my questions about their climb, encouraged Keith. He asked if I wanted to have breakfast with them when they returned from Mount Rainier, before they flew back to their homes. I did.

Several days later we connected over breakfast. While they did not reach the summit, I enjoyed learning about their adventure.

Keith and I began a steady correspondence through email and telephone calls, sharing information about our past, our current jobs and families. I loved how he talked about his children. His words made it clear that he was a papa bear. I especially enjoyed listening to him talk about his outdoor hiking adventures with his kids, as well as the pizza, taco, and spaghetti dinners he prepared for them.

Our relationship developed quickly, and our connection was a welcome joy after the past year.

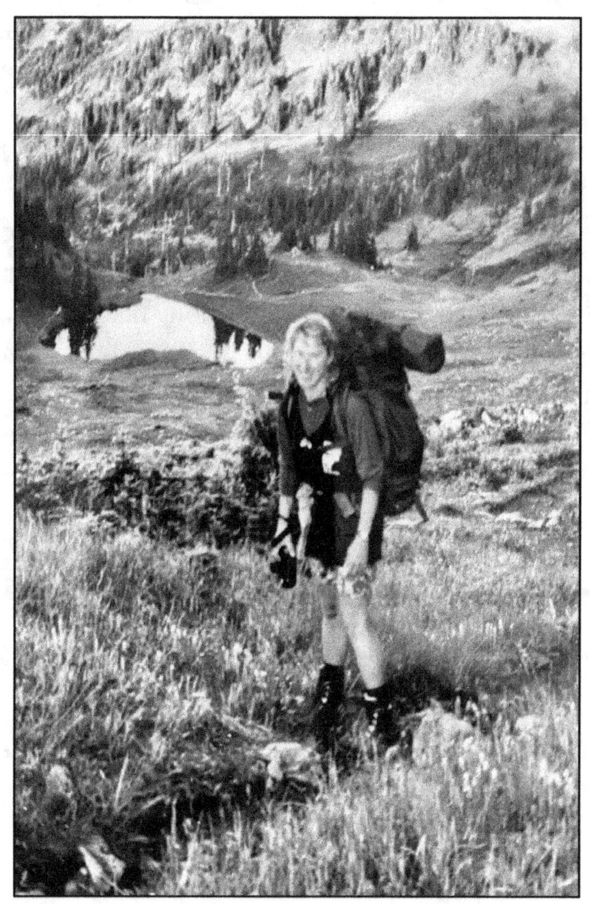

Kathleen at Heart Lake, Washington

31

A Breath of Fresh Air

I walked by him at the airport. While I remembered he was tall and thin with blonde, curly hair and freckles, I did not recall the beard. Was this a new addition? This man wore wire-rimmed glasses. Although we did not exchange photos, I knew he wore glasses. But were they wire-rimmed? I had a second of self-doubt. *Should I be heading off into the wilderness with a man I barely know?* I turned and walked by him again. A smile emerged through his rough facial hair, just as I recognized him.

After weeks of emailing and long-distance phone calls, Keith and I planned a four-day backpacking trip to Olympic National Park for early August. Time spent in the wilderness—hiking and camping— would surely determine whether we would continue this relationship. His soft-spoken manner was complemented by a subtle sense of humor, which had been evident in the playful emails we exchanged.

Initially, our meeting was awkward. *What was I doing here with a relative stranger?* But, as we drove several hours from Sea-Tac airport in the waning daylight to our first campsite, we quickly became comfortable with each other. After hours of talking and setting up camp in the dark, I fell into a peaceful slumber, my doubts dissipating into the moist, fresh mountain air.

The outdoors is where I am mentally and emotionally at my best, and I relish exploring new places. The next day, as we hiked the Sol Duc Trail along a ridge, we saw Heart Lake nestled below—our campsite for the night. The outline of the lake really did resemble a heart, surrounded by the lush greenery of the Olympic Peninsula and accented by a bright blue sky. Calling it romantic didn't capture the beauty or my strong feelings. The soft wind blew across my face, and I felt calm, safe, and wholly loved—a needed sense of belonging.

Our relationship continued to evolve after our return from the backpacking trip. Several weeks later, I met Keith's children, Sara and Sam. They were visiting their Aunt Jessica in Seattle before school started in Boulder. Keith's parents were also in town from Georgia. I had already met them during a previous visit, as Jessica and I had been friends for several years. I enjoyed their company.

The night I met Keith's children, we enjoyed a picnic dinner while listening to a summer concert at Woodland Park Zoo. We spread a large, quilted blanket on the ground near the band, and Jessica brought two comfortable outdoor chairs for her parents. I took an immediate liking to the children. Sweet, seven-year-old Sara clung closely to me all evening and hugged me when we left. Her eagerness to cling to me took me by surprise. I wondered if there was an issue at home.

In September, I flew to Boulder for a few days to see Keith's home and lifestyle firsthand. At the end of a romantic weekend, we got engaged. I was giddy with excitement.

While our relationship blossomed, my employer, a publicly traded long-term care company, was engaged in serious discussions about selling the company. It was expected that the company would be sold, and by spring 1996, the corporate offices would relocate to Kentucky.

The buyer asked me if I would move to Louisville and remain with the company as a lawyer. When I visited Louisville in the fall, I toured the offices in the late afternoon, after many of the employees had left for the day. Surprised to see clean, clutter-free, empty desks—not a single item on the surface—I asked if the offices were vacant. They were not; I was told that the company had a 'clean desk policy,' requiring employees to completely clear their desks at the end of the day.

At that moment, I knew I did not want to take the job. This rule seemed stringent and unreasonable. The majority of my coworkers had already declined to take an offer with the new entity. After some analysis, I concluded that the buyer's philosophy and corporate culture were vastly different from the beloved culture I was accustomed to. While this information helped me decide to decline the transfer to Kentucky, other factors were at play.

Amid all these changes and decisions, preliminary plans were already in place for my move from Seattle to Boulder, which was anticipated for the week after Christmas. The hurricane-like passion had some of my friends concerned, especially with all the stresses I had been dealing with that year.

When I declined the transfer to Kentucky, the acquiring company asked if I would stay until June of 1996, when they would be closing the offices in Washington and Denver. They offered me the opportunity to work at our Denver office until then, when they would pay me a handsome severance. I agreed.

Many of my friends met Keith at a goodbye dinner for me during one of his fall visits. While they were happy for me, I could tell that some of them had reservations about my decision to move and get married. They warned me about making major life decisions after such a stressful year. Although they liked Keith, they worried I might be signing up for challenging times, given the geographic move and the commitment to help raise his two young children.

While I hadn't felt this way about anyone for a long time, I had to ask myself if I was vulnerable to love as a distraction from the unrelenting anguish of dealing with Mom. Some of my friends thought so, and I had to consider their advice. Yet, a quiet voice inside insisted that the love I felt was genuine and that I was ready to raise a family.

Certainly, I was also experiencing feelings of guilt, thinking that if I was going to go through with a major move after fourteen years in Seattle, I should move closer to Mom. It wasn't the first time I felt guilt, nor the last time I would feel inadequate about decisions I made about my life, or on behalf of Mom. Since Mom was already in a nursing facility and her house had been sold, moving back to care for her in her home was not the issue. While there were many good facilities specializing in the care of Alzheimer's patients, I was now acutely aware that every home has its challenges, and family involvement is imperative to achieve consistent care.

Sometimes, when I became obsessed with moving back to the Twin Cities, I projected that my siblings thought I should, since I was single and didn't have children to take care of. No one ever said anything to me. I put this on myself, self-doubt and guilt filtering through my stoic appearance. Guilt sat on my shoulders like my thirty-five-pound backpack, heavy and relentless.

Consequently, I researched the potential for in-house healthcare legal counsel jobs in the Twin Cities during the mid-to-late 1990s, but no opportunities presented themselves. Unlike today, when many large corporations grow sizable legal departments, healthcare entities did not hire many attorneys for in-house positions back then. Most companies engaged law firms for their legal needs.

My mind was clear; I decided to move to Boulder and was excited to introduce Keith to my mom.

32

Another Thanksgiving Holiday

Keith and his children traveled to the Twin Cities to spend Thanksgiving weekend with my family. We stayed with Lori and John and their two children, Andrea and Joe, who were close in age to Sam and Sara. Family introductions on Wednesday went well. We had fun planning weekend events, including a trip to the Minnesota Children's Museum.

Our plan for Thanksgiving was to enjoy dinner at Sissy and Brian's home because they could accommodate our large group. Cheri and her family were driving down to the Twin Cities, and my brother Dan and his fiancée, Lynn, were also joining us. We were thrilled that Steve, his wife, and children would be there, making the gathering even more meaningful.

Steve had been discharged from the rehabilitation hospital in early November, so he was still adjusting to being home. We were relieved by his remarkable recovery. While he had no lingering physical limitations, his short-term memory remained a concern, setting a bittersweet tone over his return.

After a discussion with Lori, we decided to take Mom out of Tulip Place for Thanksgiving dinner. Although we worried the large crowd might be too chaotic for her, we knew how important holidays together were and that her opportunities for them in the future would be limited.

On Wednesday evening, Lori and I chatted warmly and reminisced while we prepared Mom's time-honored recipe for turkey stuffing. Lori would bake it before heading over to Sissy's home. I was thankful for the opportunity to share this tradition with her.

On Thanksgiving morning, Keith and I drove to Tulip Place while Sara and Sam stayed and played with Lori's children. When we arrived at the secure unit, I entered the code and pushed the door open. As soon as it closed, a large, well-rounded, curly-white-haired lady shuffled toward Keith.

"I'm so glad you came to see me," she said. "I've been bragging about you to my friends here, telling them that you, my dear nephew, are now an engineer. Oh! I'm so happy to see you!" She grabbed him and gave him a big hug.

Keith, a PhD engineer from Duke University, had never seen this lady before. However, he was the picture of what she described: tall, lanky, curly blonde hair, freckles, and wire-rimmed glasses. Having never been in a memory care unit before, Keith was on new ground. As I would learn was often the case with him when encountering the unexpected, he was speechless.

One of the nurses saw the interaction and started to approach the large woman who had given Keith a big hug, knowing that he was not related to her. I spoke to the boisterous woman. "Hi, I'm Kathleen, and this is Keith. He's an engineer, but he's here with me. We're visiting my mom. What a coincidence that he looks like your nephew! What's your name?"

Unconvinced by my declaration, the lady kept talking to Keith. She looked directly at him, "I'm your Aunt Lucy," she said emphatically. She studied him as the nurse took her gently by the arm, steering her away. Just then, I spotted Mom sitting at a table staring in the opposite direction from where Keith and I stood. I walked over to her, faced her, leaned down, and squeezed her body to mine.

"Hi, Mom! So nice to see you." She looked up at me, and a wide smile slowly spread across her sweet face. She was surprised, but recognized me right away.

"Hi Kathi," she said. "I didn't know you were coming! I'm so happy to see you." She tried to stand up, but her hands gripped the armrests on her chair as she fell back. She obviously didn't remember our telephone call the day before, when I told her I was in town staying with Lori.

"Sit down, Mom. I'll sit too." Mom glanced at me, and her eyes shifted to Keith with an inquiring look.

"Who are you?" She stared at Keith.

"Mom, I want to introduce you to Keith. When I visited you last month, I showed you pictures of our camping trip last summer, and I told you we're engaged to be married." She looked at me with a blank stare and then over at Keith again.

"I think…I think I remember that," she hesitated. "Hi, Keith, nice to meet you." She continued to look at him shyly.

Keith said, "Hi, Adele. Kathleen's told me so much about you. It's nice to finally meet you." He gently took her hand and held it for a few seconds.

We chatted with Mom for several minutes. She seemed to be tracking our conversation, but then wavered, looked at Keith, and said, "Who are you?"

"I'm Keith. Your daughter and I are engaged to be married."

Mom turned to me, "Really, Kathi? Oh! I'm so happy for you. I didn't know you were going to be married." She stopped as if she wanted to ask more questions, but said nothing. She looked confused and turned to Keith, then back to me, and said, "Did I show you my new home?"

"Yes, Mom. You and I take walks around your pretty home and outside in the courtyard whenever I visit. But Keith hasn't seen it yet. Should we show him?"

She hesitated for a few moments, but then said, "Yes." She tried to stand, but fell back into the chair again. Keith and I helped her up and started walking, holding on to her from both sides.

As we slowly walked around the unit, she leaned heavily on us, halting and uncertain. I said, "Mom, it's Thanksgiving today. Keith and I are here to take you to Sissy and Brian's home, where we'll all have dinner. Everyone will be there—Steve and his family too!"

She stopped walking, "Oh—I didn't know it was Thanksgiving. I guess I forgot." She paused as if trying to remember something. I wondered if a flicker of a long-ago Thanksgiving Day passed through her memory. She finally said, "Is Steve okay? I know he was in the hospital." Other fragile recollections were straining to come through, like the sun on a stormy day.

"Yes, Mom. Steve's home now. He was discharged a week ago and is living back at his home with Anne and his kids," I said.

"Oh! Oh! I'm so happy. I don't remember what happened, but I know he was very sick. It'll be so good to see him." She smiled.

After showing her "home" to Keith, we let the nurse know we were leaving. Since I had called earlier to inform the staff we would be taking Mom out for the day, they knew not to prepare dinner for her. Keith and I each took one of her arms as we walked to the car and assisted her into the back seat, buckling her in.

We arrived at Sissy's home, and the savory smells of the cooking turkey greeted us. Cheri's beautiful pumpkin and apple pies invited a taste as they rested on the counter. Mom seemed to enjoy the large gathering. She ambled around in a daze at times, managing short, coherent conversations, doing well with one-on-one chats. Earlier that morning, I had talked to Sam and Sara about my mom, explaining Alzheimer's disease. I warned them that my mom might ask their name several times. Sara stayed close to Mom, seemingly protective of her; she handed her a glass of juice when she noticed Mom didn't have a drink with her meal.

I could tell by Mom's smiling face that she was thrilled to see Steve looking and acting more like himself than he'd been in almost a year. She talked as if she remembered the course of his long illness and time in the hospital. I prompted her about the day several months earlier, when I was home and took her to see Steve at Bethesda Hospital.

"Mom, this past summer, you and I brought dinner to the hospital, and Steve was able to come outside in a wheelchair with us," I reminded her. "It was a warm, sunny day, and we had a great time eating at a picnic table on the hospital grounds. I brought hamburgers and fries from Burger King for our early dinner that day."

She nodded. It was unclear if she recalled the day. Like so often happens with memory-impaired people, they nod and agree, even if they don't remember an event. They are trying to remain a part of the family or friends' gathering, but struggle to keep up or recall names and events. Mom, normally graceful in conversations, was adept at social graces.

That day is clear in my memory. Mom started wandering away from the picnic table as I was setting the plates, silverware, and food on the tablecloth I packed for the occasion. Meanwhile, Steve made several attempts to stand up out of his wheelchair, endangering himself. I had to go after Mom, but I worried Steve wouldn't remember to sit still until I returned. It struck me as odd to be caring for two beloved family members with such different memory problems. I chuckled to myself, trying to see the glass as half full now that Steve was on a path with a better prognosis.

After the meal, Mom tired quickly. Dan took her back to Tulip Place, while the rest of us lingered to chat and play games.

I managed to sneak away every day that weekend for at least an hour or two to visit with Mom. She had many lucid moments, but they quickly dissolved and merged into long-ago memories. We reminisced, and I spoke with the nurses and nurse aides to ensure the new staff knew me and understood to call me regarding any issues.

Keith and the children left Sunday evening. My flight wasn't until Tuesday morning. I stayed another day so I could see Mom on Monday, knowing that the next month in Seattle would be busy with preparations for my move to Boulder and my new role as a stepmother.

While Keith and I did not set a specific date, we planned to marry in the summer of 1996. This lovely, poignant Thanksgiving made me realize that life is filled with sunny days and sorrowful times, and I wanted to embrace them all. As I prepared for my move to Boulder, I realized I was ready to share my life with Keith and raise a family.

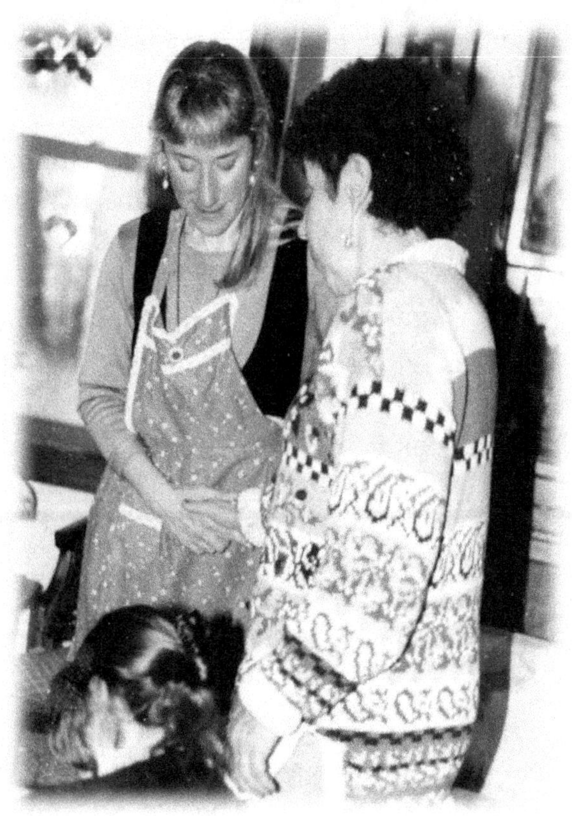

Kathleen and Mom, Thanksgiving 1995

Part V

Moves and Stages

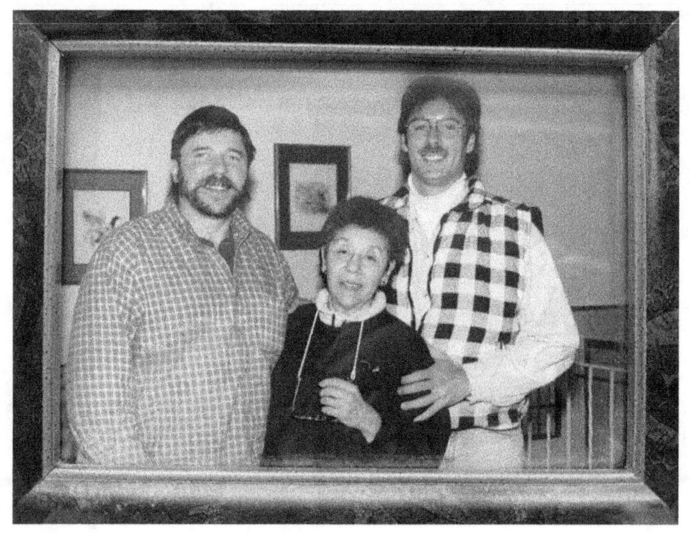

Steve, Mom, and Dan

33

Seattle to Boulder

Keith flew to Seattle on a dark, rainy December day after Christmas to help me finish packing. The movers, wearing rain gear, loaded the items we couldn't fit into my little red Nissan. The heavy drops quickly gave way to a steady drizzle, more characteristic of Seattle. Despite the chaos of the movers and boxes littering my small apartment, I was struck by how few possessions I owned. I had never been one for accumulating 'things,' preferring to spend my money on interesting events, trips, outdoor adventures, or education.

As Keith and I left Seattle and drove south, I felt a mix of excitement and anxiety. Living together, marriage, and a family life were all unknowns, and the changing weather outside mirrored the thoughts moving through my mind: heavy rain, thick clouds, a clear blue sky, and sun, with the cycle beginning again.

We spent a few days in Oregon, first visiting friends in Portland and then in Corvallis. There, at a jewelry store owned by a close friend, Keith purchased an engagement ring designed by my friend's husband. Driving across the beautiful landscapes of Oregon, Wyoming, and Colorado, we had plenty of time to talk. During the drive, we shared our expectations, dreams, and hopes for the future, discussing everything from our relationship to parenting.

Taking my impending role seriously even before we were officially married, I had bought and read books on step-parenting for insight and practical knowledge. Ultimately, my priority was not to disrupt Sam and Sara's lives. I planned to observe their routine for a few weeks, then gently introduce new ideas as I gradually integrated myself into their lifestyle. Still, beneath all my preparation, a deep anxiety lingered: would I be accepted into their home? I wasn't even sure Keith fully grasped the gravity of what I was trying to communicate.

As they had been doing, the plan was for the children to live with us for a week at a time, then spend a week with their mom and stepdad, who lived a mile away.

We discussed my mom, and Keith understood that I would travel back to Minnesota to see her as often as possible. I tried to push away the sadness, realizing that Mom would never comprehend that I was going to be married and have a family. She would be so happy for me if she could retain the memory of it.

When we arrived in Boulder late in the evening on January 3, 1996, in the middle of a snowstorm, we stopped at Stella's house—Keith's former wife and the kids' mom—to pick up the children. As it turned out, they had school in the morning, which Keith had forgotten to mention. I went to the door with Keith, feeling a mix of anticipation and nervousness. I had not yet met Stella.

The kids opened the door and gave us each a quick hug, then stood back behind Stella as she approached. They had their coats on and their suitcases by the door, ready to go. After introductions, Stella expressed gratitude that felt over-the-top, claiming the kids had been "too much" for her that week. She gave Keith a list of instructions. While discussing Sara's clarinet lessons and looking straight at me, she said to Keith. "Maybe you should have Kathleen work with Sara when she practices. I'm done with her practice sessions. I don't want to do it anymore." She waited for Keith's response. The kids stayed quiet.

"We'll see," Keith said. Nothing more. As much as I hoped this wasn't a sign of family dynamics to come, I tucked this piece of information away.

When we arrived at the house, which I'd only been to once, we unpacked our suitcases, got the kids ready for bed, and regrouped. Keith said, "I'll need you to take the kids to school tomorrow because I have an early meeting."

Caught unaware after learning the kids had school the next day, and thinking about the snow and icy weather, I said, "Why don't you call one of Sam or Sara's friends' parents and ask if they can pick up the kids in the morning? I'll have them ready, but I think that will work better since I don't know the town or the location of the school."

Keith looked at me and sighed. He called Winnie, one of the parents he knew who lived around the corner. Winnie was happy to help. She would become a good friend.

So, although we weren't yet married, I was firmly in my role as a stepparent, working my job mostly remotely from our home and traveling to my employer's Denver office twice a week.

*****

My siblings expressed happiness that I was involved with Keith and had a ready-made family, and made efforts to get to know him and his children. They all married young and had children, and they thought marriage and a family might never happen for me. There was some commonality in our lives now, which seemed to bring us closer.

Lori updated me on issues about Mom. We did not always agree on every matter, but we managed well together and tried to resolve our differences to ensure Mom was in expert hands. The nursing facility wasn't far from Lori's home, so she visited frequently. She observed Mom enjoying activities, such as listening to music in the afternoons or watching old movies. I continued to call the nursing staff at least once a week for an update on Mom, and I spoke with her directly every few days.

In the afternoon of Valentine's Day in 1996, I picked up the phone to call the facility. "Hi Mom," I said when the nurse handed her the phone. "Happy Valentine's Day! I miss you. I love you."

"Hi Kathi! It's so good to hear your voice."

I let out a breath. I hadn't realized that each time I talked to Mom, a tightness gripped my chest until I knew whether she'd recognize me.

"How are you doing, Mom? Have you been involved in any fun activities today, Valentine's Day?"

"Oh, is that what day it is?" Her voice trailed off. I imagined her looking around to see a sign that it was Valentine's Day. She sounded lucid. "Oh yes, I see on the bulletin board that there is a large red Valentine," she added.

"Mom, do you remember every year when we were little, Dad would bring us each our own little box of Valentine candies, usually my favorite, chocolate?" I waited a minute, but she didn't reply. "Did you receive the card I sent you with the big red heart on it and the box of candy I sent?"

"Yee…yes…, I think so." She hesitated. I heard her soft voice turn away from the phone as she talked to a staff member. "Did I get a card and candy from my daughter Kathi?"

I heard someone say, "Yes, Adele, it was a big, colorful card that we hung up in your room. We opened the box of chocolates right away because you wanted to share the candy with us. You're so thoughtful, Adele."

Mom turned back to the phone. "Yes, I did, Kathi. Thank you. Where're you? Are you calling from Seattle?"

"No, Mom, I moved to Boulder, Colorado, after Christmas. I sent you a postcard a couple of weeks ago." I paused to wait for her to say something. She remained silent. "Do you remember meeting Keith? You met him at Thanksgiving when we visited you. We are engaged to be married, so I moved to be with him and his children." Silence.

"Who? You mean Ed? Are you finally going to marry Ed, Kathi? Oh, I always thought you would come back to him. I was so sad when you broke up and moved to Seattle. Dad and I loved him. He's so funny, such a great guy. I'm happy for you." She sounded lucid, but she was reaching back into history.

"No, Mom. Ed and I will always love each other as friends. He met and married Dorothy a long time ago. You met Dorothy several times. We're all friends now. I know you loved him like a son, but we're not meant to be together. I'm with Keith now."

"Oh. I'm sorry. I thought you meant Ed. I don't know who Keith is."

"Keith is someone I met last year." She was silent.

"Mom, have you seen Lori lately?" I changed the subject, hoping to avoid frustrating her by talking about Keith, whom she clearly did not remember. Still, no response. "Mom, I'll come to visit you next month on your birthday," I promised, hoping to bring a bit of joy to her, even if she couldn't fully understand my current life.

"Oh, that'll be great, Kathi. I'll see you then. Bye." The phone went dead before I could say goodbye. I wondered if she felt worn out trying to summon memories. I hoped it didn't cause her undue distress. The tears came.

Trips back to St. Paul from Denver were shorter than from Seattle, and I could get away every few months to see Mom—whether it was a combined business trip or a long weekend. Whenever I visited her, we walked up and down the unit's halls and into the main part of the facility. When the weather was pleasant, we went outside.

Sometimes when I visited St. Paul, I called my Aunt Gussie to invite her to lunch, or my cousin Teresa to see if she and my aunt could meet us for dinner at Mancini's Char House, a famous steakhouse in St. Paul that we all loved. We had to plan to be out for several hours because Mom moved slowly and needed reminders to eat. Mancini's was a place where it was okay to linger. The tempting aromas from the broiled steaks, the closeness of the tables laden with freshly toasted and generously buttered white and rye toast, and Mancini's famous relish plate provided a comfortable place. We would relax, waiting for our dinner to arrive and enjoying our time together.

Conversations flowed well with Aunt Gussie. Long-term memories came easily to Mom when her sister, a captivating storyteller, shared memorable times from their childhood. Mom was bright-eyed and smiled a lot during these meals, engaging in conversations with her beloved sister. In these precious moments, I found nuggets of peace. Every time Mom smiled and laughed, a dark corner of my mind brightened. These minor pleasures were God's gift of grace and mercy.

34

Parenting

Boulder, 1996: The first year sped by like a whirlwind, a revolving door of new activities. I jumped in full speed with stepparenting, enjoying time with the kids, cooking and baking, and running with nine-year-old Sam along Boulder Creek in the crisp morning air. Afternoons were spent taking seven-year-old Sara swimming, shopping, or to plays at the local children's theater.

When the kids were with us, Keith made pizza on Friday evening, and we watched a movie or played cards. We had the children stay with us more than a week at a time because of Stella's busy schedule. This was not an issue for me, but I could see how it affected Sara.

One Saturday, Sara asked me if I knew how to make a blueberry pie. I admitted I had never made one. She said her mommy knew how to make "a very good blueberry pie." Seeing the hesitation in her eyes, I offered gently, "Why don't you call your mommy and ask for the recipe?" She paused, looked down, and in a soft whisper said she couldn't call. She would not tell me why, and I did not want to press the issue.

Sara's behavior became clear to me a few weeks later when Stella was dropping the kids off. She said, "I told the kids not to call me when they are here. I need time to myself and with James. We just got married."

Within a month of Stella telling me she did not want to hear from the kids when they were at our house, I had the opportunity to ask if she would call them every day. She had been complaining to me about Sam and Sara being "clingy" when they were with her, and that she didn't have a minute's peace. I said I loved her children, but they missed her. I offered that if they knew she was available to them—at least by phone—the clingy behavior might stop.

Much to my surprise, she started calling them every day. If I answered the phone, she would say she was "calling to give them their daily dose."

To this day, my eyes moisten thinking about what Sara said to me a week later, after talking to her mom. Smiling broadly, she exclaimed, "Kath-a-leen, my mommy said she's going to call me every day when I'm at my daddy's house!"

*****

Like the children receiving daily calls from their mom, I was trying to call my mom every few days. It gave me reassurance to hear her voice, and I hope it gave her comfort to hear mine—perhaps creating a lucid moment for her. I realized that I had been parenting my mom for several years. Now, I was adding stepparenting to my daily routine.

When I traveled to Minnesota every few months, I visited Medicaid-certified nursing facilities because Lori and I were planning ahead. While we liked several of the nurses at Tulip Place, overall, we were not impressed with the staff.

Every organization or company has a culture that permeates through the organization, mirroring the directives and attitudes of top management. Unfortunately, this company of facilities seemed to prioritize profit over resident care. While we tried to work collaboratively with the staff, I could not get over the ill feelings I had about the way they took Mom off her medications so abruptly, causing her delusions to return.

In May, I completed my remote work with my Washington employer and received a six-month severance package that allowed me to take some time off. I drove back to Minnesota, enjoying the solitude.

Lori and I had decided on placing Mom at a facility in Oakwood, Minnesota, which was reasonably close to Lori's home. Like Mom, Lori has a caregiver heart, and she had been working for a couple of years as a home health aide. Having gained insights into the care of dementia patients through her work, when she first visited the home, she asked the staff many questions, and they met her approval.

My brother Steve, while physically recovered from his illness, continued to have short-term memory difficulties. The doctors were unsure whether he would ever regain his full memory. It was not a dementia like Mom's. He didn't exhibit any signs of the progression of Alzheimer's, which often includes the breakdown of normal body functions and progressive memory decline. While he was physically back to his norm, Steve could not recall what he had done several hours earlier. His memory deficit exhibited characteristics similar to those of Drew Barrymore's character in the 2004 movie *50 First Dates*.

I enjoyed being back in Minnesota in the late spring with a flexible schedule and my own car, which gave me a sense of control I greatly needed. I picked up Steve at his home so he could visit Mom with me. She was always thrilled to see him.

"Hi, Steve, what are you doing here? It's so good to see you." Her face would soften and break into a wide smile every time we arrived for a visit. Steve always gave Mom a big hug and put an arm around her as he led her on our journeys. He, too, had a caregiver heart and was always concerned about the underdog. He would often stop people at a store or church and offer words of encouragement if he suspected they needed comfort.

We had fun times taking Mom out for short walks along the Mississippi River Boulevard near our childhood home. Sometimes we ate lunch at Perkins, a place Mom always enjoyed. If the restaurant was busy, the noise would agitate her. Shuffling when she walked, she stopped often, hesitating and looking around as if she didn't recognize her surroundings. We would remind her where we were and what we were doing. Sometimes, we had to physically lift and bend her legs to help her get into the car. Still, she managed to walk without a cane or walker.

When I dropped Steve off at his house, before getting out of the car, he would look at me and say, "Sister, I know we had a good time today. We always do when we're together. But would you please remind me what we did today? Did we see Mom?"

Regardless of how often this happened, it took me several seconds to respond with a list of what we had done that day. Despite his problems, Steve chuckled when he admitted he couldn't remember things. His laugh would end with an upbeat phrase: "It ain't easy being me, Sister, but I know God has a plan for me!"

Sometimes, I felt a little crazy spending time with two family members whom I loved dearly. Both had memory problems that changed their lives, and the lives of those who loved them.

That spring, when I left to return to Boulder, Mom had been placed on the waiting list at Oakwood. Several weeks later, Lori and I received notice that a room was available in their memory care unit, to which Mom was admitted on June 20, 1996. The physical move-out from Tulip Place to the new facility was handled by Lori, her husband, and my other siblings.

*****

When I returned to Boulder in early June, I felt refreshed from the alone time I had had driving back to Colorado. The quiet roads and wide-open spaces cleared my head in a way that had not been possible for many months. My mom's illness and her dependence on others for her care opened my eyes to life's fragility. The petty, troubling dysfunction between Keith and Stella suddenly felt like a heavy weight. I wasn't sure if I had the patience for it.

My weariness returned as soon as I was back in Boulder. Keith and I had planned to get married that summer, but I couldn't set a wedding date because of my growing doubts about his commitment to our relationship and my commitment to him.

I was often caught in the middle of disagreements between Keith and his ex-wife. Sometimes, they avoided each other and used me as a go-between rather than discuss their parenting issues together. But other times, Stella went straight to Keith and made demands that he readily complied with—demands that often involved me.

It wasn't until the fall of 1996 that I realized how low I rated on Keith's list of priorities. His children were his number one priority, as they should be. His job was number two, and his ex-wife seemed to rank higher than I did.

"She's like a business partner to me because we have kids together," he said to me. "Of course, she comes before you." That really stung. I realized he wasn't good at conflict resolution or constructive confrontation, but putting it so bluntly made me feel alone, unloved, and taken for granted.

One night, back in late winter, a couple of months into my new life in Boulder, I was working in my home office, located in the daylight basement. Keith was out at a meeting, and the kids were upstairs doing homework. I went up to check on them. I heard voices coming from a bedroom on the upper level. It was Sara and her mom.

When I walked upstairs, Stella said, "Oh, hi, Kathleen. I came by to drop some things off for Sara since she is staying here a few more days."

"Hi." I was taken aback at seeing her in my bedroom. "When did you get here? I didn't hear the doorbell ring. Did you need something in here?"

"Oh—I have a key to the house. I let myself in. I just wanted to see how you decorated the upstairs."

I was speechless.

Later, I told Keith that I wasn't comfortable with Stella having a key to our home and coming and going without notice. I asked him to reclaim the key and set new boundaries with her. Initially, he was unwilling to ask for the key or to talk to her, even though he didn't have a key to her house.

These were the times I really missed my mom. I couldn't pick up the phone and call her for comfort or guidance. Mom was always a good listener and gave wise advice. The irony of mom's ability to provide wisdom to other people, yet live for years with the unpredictability of an alcoholic, often gave me pause for contemplation.

Keith and I took a trip together that summer, a trip that was originally planned as our honeymoon. It did not repair our relationship. And even though I felt I was low on his list of priorities, when we returned from the trip, I interviewed with a law firm in Denver, where I was engaged to do part-time work while studying for the Colorado Bar exam.

I spent time with the kids, taking them on various excursions and outdoor activities. Keith had to travel to Asia for his research, and I found myself enjoying the weeks with the children, despite his absence. Months later, I would realize that I loved the children more than I loved Keith and would be very sad if I decided to sever my relationship with him, which was often on my mind.

*****

I flew back to Minnesota in early fall and again for the Thanksgiving holiday in 1996. I went alone on both visits. I am not sure if it was the move from Tulip Place to Oakwood or the natural progression of Alzheimer's, but Mom was more fragile when I visited. The literature on Alzheimer's disease discusses that changing rooms, homes, or daily routine can adversely affect the person with dementia, increasing the pace of the disease's progress.

Shortly after Mom entered the Oakwood Memory Care unit, she started to have problems with falls. By autumn, she was using the assistance of a Merry-Walker to ambulate. This device combines the parts of a walker and a wheelchair. It features a safety belt for added security and a seat to sit, allowing individuals to walk as far as they can and rest as needed without the risk of falling. Today, however, Merry Walkers may or may not be used for people with severe cognitive impairments because they are enclosed in a frame from which a person cannot easily release themselves. Depending on the resident's assessment and cognition, it may be considered a restraint and subject to strict regulations prohibiting restraints in facilities.

Oakwood turned out to be a good choice for Mom. The not-for-profit facility was part of a large faith-based national nursing facility company. The corporate headquarters was on the East Coast. They enjoyed the fruits of a good reputation. My siblings and I found the staff to be caring, warm, and friendly.

The facility was not as beautifully maintained and manicured as Tulip Place, but the staff was far more approachable and compassionate. Oakwood did not have an all-female memory care unit like the one Mom had resided in at Tulip Place, but it didn't seem as important anymore, especially as Mom declined. Based on the unit's circular design and the caring staff, I trusted that this home closely monitored its residents, particularly regarding interactions between female and male residents.

During and after my visits to Minnesota at the end of 1996, Lori and I worked with the staff to manage Mom's decline. Mom was losing weight, and we made sure she was getting the necessary calories to maintain her weight. While medically stable, she did not eat well unless someone fed her, so we requested the staff assist her at mealtime. Whenever I visited, I tried to arrive at mealtime so I could help her. I would call the facility in advance, so they could plan accordingly. It made me feel better to be able to help in some small way.

Mom appeared more sedated during one of my visits in the fall. I spoke with the facility's medical director about making appropriate medication adjustments. If I wasn't in town for the quarterly care meetings, the facility provided me with a call-in number so I could attend via telephone conference call and keep current on Mom's care.

While I was in frequent contact with Lori and the facility, events and emotions continued to change rapidly, particularly with Keith and our life in Colorado. The changes would lead to a much different outcome than I had imagined when I moved there with the intent to marry Keith.

35

Know What You Can Control

My worry about Mom's condition gave way to bittersweet moments with her, on the phone and in person, as she descended further into her memory banks. Current times and events clearly escaped her, but she still had moments of clarity that offered encouragement. Our conversations were shorter as she struggled to find words. Sometimes I simply held the phone, listening to her breathing.

Meanwhile, during the same period in Boulder, my days became a series of emotional shifts, marked by happy, serene moments with Keith exploring the abundant hiking and ski trails in Colorado, and the devastating chasm of emotional distance at home. It became increasingly apparent that Keith and I bonded over our love of the outdoors and travel. However, life could not be sustained as a series of outdoor adventures, ignoring the glaring communication issues between us.

Our communication styles were vastly different. Keith often withdrew into silence during disagreements. This left me feeling isolated and unheard, stirring up memories of my childhood, when we often kept silent rather than resolving issues at home.

Throughout my life, I had intermittently sought individual professional counseling and Adult Children of Alcoholics (ACOA) group meetings to deal with issues from my dad's chronic drinking. When I was young, as is common in children of alcoholics, I thought that if I was well-behaved, got good grades, babysat my siblings, and helped around the house, I would make Dad proud, and he would fulfill his annual promise to quit drinking.

When I was in high school, I realized how futile these recurring promises were, so I left home after graduation. I knew by then that you cannot change another person's behavior; they have to want to change it themselves.

Nonetheless, here I was trying to resolve our differences and create a happy future with Keith. We had discussed having a child, which had become increasingly important to me. I recognized the need to consider my options as I approached a pivotal point in my life.

I had wonderful friends who were always willing to listen to me. While supportive, after hearing my sadness and identifying my stress level, many suggested I leave the relationship. What would Mom have said? I wondered. Oh, how I wish she could have meaningful conversations with me. The saving grace was that she would not have to agonize over her daughter's depressive state.

Finally, during one teary-eyed session with my therapist in Boulder, whom I had been seeing for months, I said, "Just tell me how I can fix this! What can I do to make things right with Keith?"

She looked into my teary eyes and was silent for what seemed like several minutes before she replied, "Kathleen, you can't fix this. It takes two. You are the only one in the relationship who thinks there is a problem." She paused. "You have to decide whether you want to continue to live with Keith's view of the world, or move on."

Wow! Hearing the truth was a turning point for me. The relief I felt was like a tidal wave sweeping away my angst and indecision. I had tried to influence change in my dad when I was young, and now I was doing the same thing with Keith. As the realization settled in, my body relaxed for the first time in months. The path forward was clear and within my control.

In February 1997, I had taken and passed the Colorado Bar exam intending to make Colorado my permanent home. I liked Boulder's charm and enjoyed the thriving social life, but now I was considering a move to start fresh. Still, I drove around looking for houses to rent, thinking that staying in Boulder would allow me to see the kids, even if Keith and I split.

I started networking and looking for jobs, but the reality was that staying in Boulder wasn't ideal for my career. I began calling my legal and healthcare colleagues across the country to see if they had insights into corporate counsel openings. I focused on Minnesota because of Mom, as well as Washington and Colorado—the two states where I had a license to practice law.

Then, one colleague reminded me of two national nursing home companies headquartered in New Mexico. I was familiar with Horizon Healthcare because they had offered me a job in September of 1995, nearly two years earlier. Back then, a recruiter flew me to Albuquerque for an interview. The same month I was offered the job, Keith proposed to me. I had chosen Keith and a family over the job and my career.

Sun Healthcare Group was another long-term care company in Albuquerque, and one colleague shared that they were looking to hire an attorney. After interviews in early spring, I accepted a job offer with Sun. Because this was the second job offer in Albuquerque in less than two years, I knew I was meant to be in New Mexico.

I told Keith in mid-April that I would be leaving. Tears welled in his eyes. "But I wanted to be married," he said. I know he did. I believed he wanted a wife and someone to help with the children and finances. But I did not feel loved or special.

"Yes, I know you do," I said. "But I'm not sure that it matters if it's me or someone else." Was he oblivious to this? I tried to explain my feelings to no avail. He really didn't understand how I felt—nor did he refute my perceptions.

*****

Once I had accepted the job, I went to visit Mom. It was May 1997—another spring visit. The orange and red tulips were maturing, and the yellow daffodils and lush green grass showed their brightness after the late winter snows and the April rain. Mom still met me with delight at first sight each time I visited, but the recognition waned as we talked and she meandered around the unit in her walker.

I shared the changes in my life with Mom. I told her about the turmoil in my relationship with Keith, expressed my sadness that it had ended, but also acknowledged that it was the best decision for me. I know she didn't comprehend what I was saying, but there were glimmers of recognition, and one moment of what I believed to be a look of genuine concern for me. I knew she was trying to listen despite her declining mental capabilities.

When I visited the facility, I usually reviewed the survey documents, which were available at the front desk. I remained satisfied that the caregivers at Oakwood strove to provide good care. The home had no significant deficiencies, and the staff were more welcoming than they ever were at Tulip Place.

My time with Mom brought me some peace of mind. I believed she was in good hands at this facility. Each time I visited, they asked me questions about Mom and her life. They were genuinely interested in her past and commented on the pictures we posted, as well as the small treasures we brought and left for her. Their kindnesses pierced my heart and soothed my inner conflict.

*****

In June, Keith and I sat down with Sam and Sara to share the news of my move. We remained cordial, even enjoying a few final activities together. The weeks leading up to my departure were filled with packing, visiting, and last-minute outings. Keith planned a vacation with the kids for the week the movers were scheduled to arrive.

Surprisingly, Keith's parents visited for a few days to help me pack and say goodbye; they even took me out to dinner the night before I left. Given the chaos of their son's relationship with his ex-wife, they admitted they were surprised I had stayed as long as I did. While I didn't necessarily need their approval, their kindness validated my decision. I hugged them tightly before stepping into my car the next morning.

Keith and I kept in touch after I moved, and I spoke with the children a few times. He even visited me once in Albuquerque. Soon, though, he began dating again, and our contact ultimately came to an end. At that time, I decided to stop reaching out to the children because I was worried it might confuse them. Despite that choice, I deeply missed their company, their curious minds, and their lively spirits.

Kathleen A. Hessler

36

Heading to Albuquerque

As I drove south to my new life in Albuquerque in late July, the wide-open spaces filled me with anticipation for a future full of promise. As is often the case in making major life decisions, once I was certain about leaving Keith, the heavy clouds lifted. It felt like looking up at an endless blue sky, like the skies of New Mexico. I had a blank poster board onto which I could paint a grand adventure.

Back in the fall of 1995, when I flew to Albuquerque to interview for a job I ultimately declined, I spent three unforgettable days in New Mexico. During the visit, I drove north to Santa Fe, eager to explore the vast expanses of land. It was my first time in the state. My memories are vivid: walking around the plaza in Santa Fe, breathing in the scent of roasted green chiles, and savoring the delicious piñon nuts. I sauntered through the quaint alleys and streets, appreciating the old adobe buildings and window-shopping while admiring creative, colorful jewelry in turquoise, coral, and jade. I thought of Mom and her love of Mexican and Hispanic culture. She would have enjoyed what the Southwest has to offer.

*****

Now, nearly two years later, as I drove through Colorado greenery into the bright blue sky of New Mexico, my eyes blurred. I realized that I suppress my sorrow about missing and sharing things with my mom. I reflected on her trip to Mexico to visit me in the summer of 1990, recalling her excitement as she planned the trip. I thought of her delight in the mariachi music, the folklorico dancers, and tasty margaritas. I remembered how happy she was dancing with Rodney.

Even though Mom was still alive, she was leaving us bit by bit. The constant underlying bereavement from her slow decline stayed with me. The realization tore at my heart and drenched my spirit. I thought about how fun it would have been if she had ridden with me as I moved south from Boulder to Albuquerque. We could have taken in the rural countryside, the breathtaking landscapes, and the Hispanic and Native American cultures together.

I drove only half a day, stopping in Taos at the historic Sagebrush Hotel where I planned to stay the night. After checking in and walking the grounds, I went to the hotel's restaurant, whose decor is rich in cultural artifacts. I sat alone, admiring the Native paintings on the walls, while savoring a margarita and toasting to Mom's vibrant spirit, experiencing a mix of smiles and tears, happy memories and sad ones. Yet, feelings of independence and adventure stirred. I recalled the raw beauty of the watermelon-colored Sandia Mountains at sunset, visible from nearly anywhere in Albuquerque.

As I continued my journey the next day, guilt played on my mind. I imagined a conversation with Mom. "Would you want me to move back to Minnesota to be near you?" I asked.

I heard her familiar voice whisper back, "No, my daughter, live your life, follow your dreams—that is what I have wanted for you. You have given so much already. I love you." It was then that I realized each new memory of my life's journey is but a continuing connection with her.

Driving the sparsely populated roads with time to think, I wondered how much Mom grasps about her life as she slowly slips away. Does she have a sense of peace or calm? Does she experience joy or happiness during lucid moments? If she feels sadness or depression, how long do these emotions last?

Not truly understanding her level of awareness and emotional state haunted me. The unknown pressed heavily on my heart. I wanted to believe that the staff's kindness and the nurses' competency provided a comfortable routine. And knowing that she was not in physical pain, I wanted to believe she was not suffering.

My final thoughts as I rolled into Albuquerque that evening were: Am I honoring my mom by living my life, as she frequently told me to do? Was she asking me to promise her that?

Her words echoed: "Live your life. I will live vicariously through you." Absorbing the glow of the western sun on the mountains, I affirmed my promise to live fully and brightly for her.

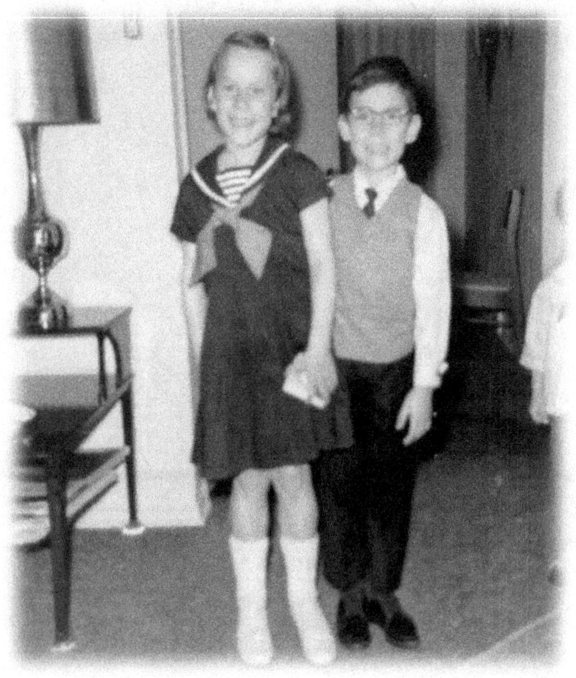

Kathleen and Dan with Lori peeking in, circa 1964

37

Financial Facts and Family Fractures

As co-conservators for Mom under Minnesota law, Lori and I were required to file an annual report with the court each March detailing how we spent money from Mom's conservatorship account, which was in both of our names.

One section of the document, called the "Personal Well-Being Report," required us to verify changes in Mom's living conditions. This included an evaluation of the care she received at the facility. We had to attest to her physical and mental well-being, any antipsychotic medications she was taking, and hospital admissions that year.

Finally, to complete these responsibilities, we were required to state the basis for our findings. For example, we included information from the medical records and documented the approximate number of visits we made to see Mom, as well as the care conferences we attended. Throughout this process, we relied on Ken Rhodes for guidance and assistance with filing these reports.

Lori and I both wrote checks from Mom's conservatorship account. Lori usually paid the facility fees, and I paid Mom's health insurance. Also, Lori used the money for clothes and other necessities for Mom. She ensured Mom was always impeccably dressed, honoring Mom's sense of style by matching shoes and earrings with her outfits. Lori resembled Mom in this way; she was meticulous in her dress and in maintaining her home and garden. Unlike Mom, who tended to run late, Lori was always punctual.

Sometimes, Lori wrote checks when she bought gifts for a grandchild's birthday, signing a card on Mom's behalf, which Mom would have approved. Per Ken's suggestion, Lori also paid herself a small conservatorship fee of about forty dollars per month. While conservator companies may bill from fifty to several hundred dollars an hour, families aren't usually paid for their services without court approval and documentation. Lori spent many hours taking care of Mom and used gallons of gas, so I was glad Ken approved a nominal monthly fee. Occasionally, I reimbursed myself for long-distance calls to the facility.

In late winter 1997, before my move to Albuquerque that summer, a pivotal moment occurred. After years of spending my own money traveling home and taking vacation days or time off without pay, I asked Lori's opinion about reimbursing me from the conservatorship account for one airplane ticket home. I believed this was a valid expense under conservatorship rules, although I had planned to confirm with Ken. I was trying to set a time and date to return to Minnesota for a care conference.

I was alarmed by the anger my simple question triggered in Lori and my brother Dan. They both sent me letters filled with misunderstandings. I had not spoken directly to Dan in months, so it was unexpected to hear from him, especially through a critical letter. At that time, long-distance calls were expensive, so we rarely spoke. Lori usually communicated with both of us. I am not certain what she conveyed to Dan.

In his letter, which was all capitalized as if he were yelling at me, he wrote that he thought my life was a walk in the park compared to his. *How does he know what is going on in my life?* We rarely talked. While we always hugged each other in greeting when we gathered for holidays or family meetings, those times were often too chaotic to have meaningful discussions. He seemed influenced by Lori, and both appeared to believe my life was stress-free. Their accusations hurt and left me doubting myself. Dan implied I was taking his inheritance, suggesting a misunderstanding about the money in a separate account in my name.

To provide context to our financial responsibilities, when Lori and I became co-powers of attorney for Mom in 1992, Ken Rhodes had advised us on care and estate planning, with a focus on Mom's future need for Medicaid. Ken understood the importance of setting aside money for expenses that Medicaid does not cover. He advised Lori, as co-power of attorney with me, to gift a certain amount of Mom's money to me each month for about twelve to eighteen months. Ken told us that he had discussed this idea with Mom when he worked with her to execute the power of attorney documents.

We agreed with Ken's advice and followed through with this directive. Since I was the only single sibling and a co-agent with Lori, Ken advised me to open the bank account in my name, keeping the money in the immediate family.

Furthermore, Ken stated that he had discussed estate planning with Mom. In keeping with Dad's previous wishes, expressed while he was alive, Mom also hoped to leave each of us a monetary inheritance. Ken said people can gift limited amounts of money to others each year without tax consequences. Then, if the gifted amounts of money were given thirty-six months—called the look-back period—prior to the person applying for Medicaid, those funds were *not* included in the assets taken into account for eligibility. Today, the general rule for the look-back period is sixty months, or five years. Ken advised us that if Mom passed before the money was used for her care, I should divide it equally among my siblings. Thus, it was not unreasonable for any of my siblings to consider this money as a possible inheritance.

In Minnesota, the Medicaid program determines eligibility for nursing home care based on a person's assets (less than $3,000) and income. A person must contribute most of their income to the cost of nursing home care, such as Social Security, investments, pensions, and other assets. The program allows the Medicaid recipient to keep a small allowance for personal needs, such as hair salon or clothing.

I had pristine records of the account Ken advised me to open. I had neither used the money nor mixed it with personal funds. It was in the bank, earning interest. In the event we didn't need this money for Mom's care, per Ken's advice, I would divide it equally among my siblings when Mom died.

Given her letter, Lori may have believed that I was spending or intended to spend the money in this account. Dan's letter suggested the same. This could have been easily resolved if we had discussed the issue. I had the bank statements for reference. We were not talking about large sums of money. Unfortunately, Lori would not return my calls, making a resolution impossible at that point.

While I was sympathetic to Lori's responsibilities with Mom and her apparent stress level, I needed to help her understand that I did not use that account. I tried to forget their hurtful letters, but it was difficult. Her unwillingness to discuss it intensified my sense of isolation.

Not understanding her real concerns, I wrote a long letter to Lori detailing responses to her assertions, and I attached copies of the bank statements. A couple of weeks later, my heart pounded when I saw the large unopened manila envelope in my mailbox with the words "return to sender" penned in Lori's handwriting. I felt a surge of emotional pain.

I did not send a copy of this letter to Dan because he told me he didn't want to hear back from me. In retrospect, I should have sent him a copy of the letter anyway. I was exhausted and didn't feel I had the energy to communicate with him.

Still, loving memories of caring for my younger brother, who was two grades behind me, spilled forth. I remembered his first day of kindergarten. It may have been his fifth birthday, since he turned five the first week of September. After Mom dropped him off at school, a teacher came to my second-grade classroom and took me to see Danny, who was crying. I removed his dark-framed glasses and wiped his eyes, hugging him. I told him my classroom was just down the hall, and I would come back to check on him again that morning. We had just moved into a new neighborhood, so there were many changes to adjust to.

Other memories came to mind as I felt a strong sense of family loss. I recalled Dan, Steve, and me peddling our bikes home from their Little League baseball games on hot summer evenings as Mom directed.

After Dan graduated from the Brown Institute of Broadcasting and took a job in Austin, Minnesota, I found comfort in listening to him on the local radio station while attending nursing school in Rochester.

*****

Unfortunately, financial issues, regardless of amount, cause many conflicts in families during illness and at the time of death. Looking back, I realized the importance of communications as we navigated these challenges. Perhaps I could have done a better job of keeping my siblings informed about this account, its purpose, and status. This situation had me rattled. These uncertainties prompted me to seek advice from Ken, our long-time advisor.

I sent copies of my siblings' letters to Ken. I also sent him a copy of the letter I wrote to Lori, then called to get his perspective and advice, since he knew our family well. He confirmed my thoughts—that my siblings' words clearly showed they thought my life was worry-free. He shared that none of my siblings, not even Lori, understood that while I was living away, I put in many hours dealing with issues that arose with Mom and traveled back and forth multiple times a year—all at my expense. Ken consoled me, telling me that my parents would be proud of me for what I have accomplished and for the work I am doing to help Mom.

Then Ken offered his opinion that my siblings were envious of me because I didn't have the day-to-day burdens that they likely felt living close to Mom. This did not surprise me, but I looked at my siblings and their beautiful children and families and thought they were blessed. At times, I envied them. They had each other close by to celebrate special events and holidays and to lend support. I made the decision to live away years ago, driven by my love of travel and the outdoors. Also, the sad memories of growing up were difficult for me to completely let go of, and I was reminded of them each time I was home.

Ken had no real advice on how to handle this situation if Lori and Dan were unwilling to engage in conversation. He said he would call

Lori to discuss the truth with her and to see if there was something he could do to help. I felt better after talking to Ken. The pain dissipated slowly over the next several months. As often happened in our family, issues were buried or ignored without direct communication. On another day, another time, we would become amiable and loving with each other again, regardless of whether the issue was resolved.

In recent years, Dan and I have had fruitful conversations, and he has expressed his trust in me. He said he didn't recall Mom's money situation—that he wasn't privy to the information. But he remembers talking to Lori and writing a letter, for which he apologized. He said he was going through a particularly difficult time back then, and he regrets writing it.

When I come into conflict with my siblings, I try to examine my actions to see what I could have done to avoid it or resolve it. Although it's not easy to know what my siblings are going through at any given time, I try to extend grace, and hope they will do the same for me.

38

Nursing Facility Challenges

My last visit to Minnesota before I moved to Albuquerque was in May 1997. Tensions with Lori were obvious, but she would not discuss her concerns. She had returned my unopened letter weeks before. The years of caring for Mom continued to demand our time and attention as we navigated our active lives.

For me, however, the sustained inner turmoil continued to cause distress. I loved my sister and cherished the bond we shared. I continued to reach out to her, confident that our shared love for our mother would prevail and bring us together again—sooner, rather than later.

In the Twin Cities, Ed, Dorothy, and my friend Molly—who knew Mom and my family well—were a great support. After tough days visiting Mom at the facility, they would listen to me over dinner. And they stayed in touch when I was back in Albuquerque.

June 1997 marked the one-year anniversary of Mom's admission to Oakwood. She resided in the memory care unit, despite her decreasing ability to walk. In May, when I visited, she was ambulating fairly well with the Merry Walker, but by autumn 1997, at sixty-two years old, her ability to walk was rapidly deteriorating.

*****

Still at work in Albuquerque, I was finishing up a meeting in my office when my phone rang. My colleagues waved as they left my office. I barely said hello before Lori blurted out, "They want to move Mom out of memory care today."

"Slow down, Lori," I said. "Did you say the facility wants to move Mom today?"

"Yes," she said. "They're planning to move her to a wing outside the memory care unit." She sounded distressed.

"Did you receive a written notice from Oakwood that they planned to transfer her?" I asked. "I haven't."

"No, this is the first I've heard of their plan. Can they do this?"

"No, not if you didn't give them permission," I said. "Under the regulations, without permission from you or me, as Mom's legal representatives, the facility must provide us with written notice of its intent to change Mom's room, or transfer her to another unit in the facility. While there are exceptions, they can't relocate her without our consent or advance written notice."

"Well, they said she doesn't meet the criteria to be in the memory care unit anymore because she's not a wandering risk," Lori said. "But I don't want her to move. I really like the staff, and Mom has settled in so well."

Previously, Lori and I had discussed Mom's decreasing ability to ambulate and the likelihood that she would have to move out of the memory care unit in the future. Moving any person with declining memory is difficult—for them and their family. We had come to trust and rely on the staff in the unit.

After talking with Lori, I called the facility administrator and unit director. I explained that while I understood Mom was no longer a wandering risk and did not need the secure unit, our family had grown accustomed to the staff. We knew a move was inevitable, but we were not prepared for an abrupt change to new faces and surroundings.

The administrator agreed to work with us. Because the situation had changed and Mom's bed was no longer needed, she was able to remain in memory care. He explained that the facility was expanding its long-term care unit, which is where Mom would eventually be transferred. Most residents on that floor needed help with all daily activities, and many had little to no communication skills. He confirmed that we would receive a thirty-day notice before her move and suggested we begin to familiarize ourselves with the staff on that unit.

Although one can find quality nursing facilities, it's not a replacement for the ongoing presence of family. The staff will often listen to and work with families who communicate their needs and concerns to the staff, and who genuinely want to be part of the care.

When I visited Oakwood, I continued building relationships with the staff so they would recognize me when I called the facility. Mom could no longer speak in full sentences, so phone conversations ended, but I felt a strong connection to the staff.

We posted family photos of important events on Mom's bulletin board so she could see them. Lori also brought in her children's art projects and drawings. Sharing Mom's pictures and stories with the staff helped them understand what her life was like before her illness. They were sincere when they asked questions about her life. They played Mom's favorite music during the day and at night to soothe her.

When I visited Mom, I played some of the big band cassettes and reminisced about evenings we spent listening to The Swinging Ambassadors at live venues. The Kahler Hotel in Rochester was one of those places. It was also where I balanced trays as a cocktail waitress while attending nursing school. Mom and Dad visited me there several times when the band was scheduled to play. Back then, their music filled the smoky lounge as Mom smiled and swayed, enjoying herself as she sipped a margarita or a glass of wine. Sometimes, she was able to get Dad out on the dance floor.

During the two years after nursing school, when I lived and worked in the Twin Cities, I took Mom to see them, as well as other bands, at Diamond Jim's Supper Club in Lilydale and other venues. Mom never got to hear that in 2011, after over thirty years in the business, The Swinging Ambassadors were inducted into the Minnesota Music Hall of Fame.

While Mom was no longer able to participate in conversations during my visits, she would look at me and listen. Sometimes a hint of recognition would show in her eyes before they went blank again.

I had an old postcard of the band. I showed it to her. I tried not to be discouraged, but I liked to believe she could understand some of what I was saying. So, I continued to share stories from the past, as well as new stories about my life. Sometimes I read to her. She always enjoyed good magazine articles.

*****

As a conservator, I had access to Mom's medical records. I would periodically request copies so I could review the care and medications she received. The legal representative of a loved one has the right to access and obtain copies of the medical records. In May 1997, when I visited her, I should have requested monthly copies of her daily records. I knew that with my move to Albuquerque and starting a new job, I would not be able to return to Minnesota for many months.

It wasn't until late October that I returned for a visit, about a month after I spoke to the administrator about the transfer issue. This was the longest stretch I had gone without seeing her in prior years.

Since it had been over five months, I drove directly to the facility upon my arrival in the Twin Cities. When I walked into Mom's room, I saw her lying in bed, curled up on her right side in the fetal position. She was sleeping, with light snores coming from the bed.

I touched her hand lightly, and she moved, then grimaced as if she were in pain. I tried to raise her arm to my face. Her arm was bent at the elbow and would not straighten out. I tried to do the same with her other arm and legs. She was bound with contractures in all four extremities.

Looking around the dimly lit room, I took a deep breath. Questions raced through my mind. Where was the range of motion chart? Had the staff neglected these exercises? My worry heightened. This was not right. This was not a classic progression of Alzheimer's disease if she were getting proper passive range of motion exercises.

39

Contractures

I took a few minutes to compose myself. I felt hot as my anger swelled and my blood pressure rose. I stared at my mom's hand, twisted into an unnatural angle. I wanted to shout: *How did you let this happen to my mom? Basic nursing 101 core principles state that passive range of motion (PROM) exercises are a standard part of the care for the immobile patient.*

It broke my heart to see Mom's twisted body. Contractures are painful and develop from decreased movement of muscles and joints, leading to muscle and tendon tightening and joint shortening and stiffening. Her four extremities were inflexible, and her hands curled inward. She grimaced with pain when I tried to lift her arm or untwist her fist to hold her hand.

It was clear that the staff wasn't doing PROM exercises. In Alzheimer's, as the brain atrophies, it ceases to tell the body what to do. Mom's brain no longer told her to move, to stretch, or to turn. In later stages of the disease, the risk of contractures of all four extremities increases as people lose both gross and fine motor skills.

I was shocked by how quickly Mom was spiraling downward, yet, I believed these contractures could have been prevented to a large extent. Preventative measures should have been taken by the nursing staff. These included positioning Mom in bed or a chair with the right mattresses and support equipment, such as blankets, cushions, wedges, and pillows.

When I walked into the room, the first thing I noticed was that Mom's head was hyperextended, with no form of support under her neck. There were no cushions between her legs; lying in the fetal position, her two thin legs rested on top of each other. Two flat pillows should have been placed between the legs: one at the knee upwards and one extended beyond the foot. A rolled blanket would have provided support and comfort under her arm.

Many medical directors, if advised of Mom's resistance to PROM efforts, would have ordered physical and occupational therapy consults to assess her and to provide staff with guidance on preventing and treating contractures. I was fairly certain that the nursing staff had not consulted the medical director.

I left the room and went to see the director of nursing. I liked her and had gotten to know her well over the year. Together, we went to my mom's room, where I pointed out how poorly she was positioned in bed. I drew the DON's attention to Mom's stiff joints and her visible contractures. My voice was curt as I tried to control my anger. She could tell I was upset. I did not want to discuss the issues in Mom's room. Instead, I asked her to get my mother's medical record so we could discuss this privately. I walked ahead of her to the conference room, afraid to speak until my anger subsided. I shut the door and waited, my heart pounding in my chest.

I knew how to navigate the nursing home's medical records, so when the DON brought in Mom's chart, I took it from her. I turned to the flow sheets where the nurse aides check boxes to document whether they performed PROM exercises. I reviewed the narrative nursing notes, looking for weekly updates or for any unusual incidents. These records, however, revealed nothing about the development of Mom's contractures.

Yet, the boxes on the flow sheets were all checked, indicating that my mom had supposedly received PROM exercises twice daily for the past several weeks. I was dismayed. I knew this was false reporting, because if the staff were consistently performing this treatment, my mother's contractures would not be so severe—or even developed at all.

"I am concerned that these exercises are not being done," I said, trying to stay composed. "It appears the staff may be documenting care that they are not doing. I don't believe my mother would be in this condition if the exercises were being performed consistently."

The DON took the chart from me and scanned through the flow sheets. She said nothing. Although there was no excuse for this, I wondered whether the staff lacked experience with PROM exercises, since the unit was designed for mobile dementia residents. Maybe they did not understand the importance of these drills. Yet, these were core principles in the nursing care of immobile patients. All nursing staff should have been aware of the risk for contractures in Mom as she became less mobile. More importantly, they should have been trained on how to prevent them.

"I want to see the administrator and speak to him about this. I want the medical director to examine her and to order physical and occupational therapy immediately," I demanded.

The DON said everyone had gone home for the day, but she would call the medical director. She said, "I will definitely ask him to see her, but I don't know if your mom will qualify for occupational or physical therapy since she is now on Medicaid. You do know that she recently qualified for Medicaid, don't you?"

Frustrated, I responded, "Yes, I am aware that my mom is on Medicaid insurance. But, my understanding is that Minnesota Medicaid covers certain therapies annually for people with cognitive impairments or dementia-related diagnoses." I paused for a minute, but the DON said nothing, so I continued, "It would have been helpful if you had informed Lori and me about Mom's contractures earlier, so we could've made timely, informed decisions for her care. If Medicaid doesn't cover physical or occupational therapies, we can decide whether we will pay," I said, trying to keep my tone calm.

"Okay, okay," the director answered. "I'll research this and call the medical director in the morning."

In the meantime, I asked her to help me reposition Mom. While moving her to a more comfortable position, I examined my mom's back and buttocks to ensure there were no pressure sores developing. This is another area of concern for the immobile resident. Thankfully, she had none. Once we finished in Mom's room, I asked the DON to update the care plan instructions for positioning measures, using appropriate pillows, blankets, or wedges to support Mom's stiff, twisted body. I said I would be back in the morning to further discuss this and expected to see orders for the therapies.

We had been so happy with the care here. The staff had always been reassuring and attentive when I visited, and they were cooperative and responsive when I called. They listened attentively when I asked questions and seemed genuinely interested in Mom.

When I left the facility, I drove over to Lori's house even though I was staying with friends. Lori's family was finishing dinner. We sat in her kitchen and talked. I told Lori I was shocked to see the extent of the deterioration of Mom's body. She said it was probably more of a shock to me since I hadn't seen her in five months, but that she had noticed it too.

I asked Lori why she hadn't told me about Mom's change in condition, since it seemed to have taken a drastic turn for the worse. She said she thought it was the normal process of Alzheimer's disease. Yes, and no, I told her. I explained how the rapidity and severity of Mom's contractures tell the story of the facility not performing PROM on Mom twice daily as directed in the nursing care plan.

Like me, Lori was surprised because she thought the facility was taking good care of Mom, despite the recent issue about the room change. I agreed with Lori, but said it is an ever-vigilant job to ensure Mom is receiving proper treatments and medications. She agreed, and although she visited Mom frequently, she didn't realize preventive measures should have been implemented.

Once I calmed after seeing Mom that afternoon, I told Lori that I thought the certified nurse aides (CNAs) were attempting to perform PROM exercises. "I suspect Mom screams out or becomes agitated when they work with her, and then they stop trying," I said.

According to the quarterly care conference notes in the medical record, Mom continued to experience periods of agitation and screaming episodes, despite the medications she received to control these outbursts. However, her agitation was no excuse for the staff to document that they performed the exercises. I told Lori that I would find out the facts from the nurses and aides the next morning.

I arrived early and spoke to the administrator, the medical director, and the physical and occupational therapists. Indeed, Minnesota Medicaid paid for maintenance therapies for patients with my mom's condition—at least back then. Today, Medicaid rules may differ. The medical director ordered the treatments to start promptly.

That morning, I introduced myself to the aides who had been assigned to my mother's care in the previous days and weeks—a few remembered me from prior visits, as I did them. I wanted to understand the challenges they were facing and foster a collaborative environment. I asked what time of day they performed the PROM exercises with Mom and whether they had any difficulties working with her. Each one paused before answering.

Almost everyone said, "We try to do the exercises with Adele, but she screams loudly and pulls away. It's hard to work with her when she is upset, so when she becomes agitated, we have to stop."

While I acknowledged that my mom can be challenging, I emphasized the importance of following through on the care plan and notifying their supervisor immediately if they are unable to complete a care plan directive. Finally, I let them know, gently but firmly, that falsely recording something in the medical record, even if it involves checking a box that indicates something was done when it wasn't, is a serious issue. They should never document that they did something when they didn't complete the order.

I then discussed how to work with my mom. I asked each aide again what time of day they tried to perform the exercises. The common answer was in the morning, after Mom ate breakfast, but before her bath. I advised them, based on my review of the record and my observation of my mom, that she was generally more agitated in the mornings and late evenings. I told them that my mom is the calmest after lunch when she goes down for a nap. I asked the CNA assigned to Mom that day if she would meet me in Mom's room after lunch.

After Mom finished eating and was settling in for a nap, I demonstrated how to perform the exercises. I said it was important to schedule PROM when she was least agitated and her body was relaxed. Every day that week, I arrived in the morning and stayed until early to mid-afternoon or evening, talking with and teaching the staff how to exercise Mom.

She received physical and occupational therapy five days a week for two weeks, then three days a week for several more weeks, with a gradual tapering off of the sessions. The therapists provided splints for her hands and wrists, and the nurse aides became adept at providing the exercises. The facility kept me informed, and I spoke with the nurses regularly.

I requested Mom's records and tracked her progress monthly. I reviewed the treatment notes and was pleased to see that she regained some flexion and extension following the intensive therapy. The notes reflected improved staff awareness and consistent treatments.

Reversing contractures doesn't come easily, or at all. One of the goals is to loosen the joints and ease the pain. The medical director ordered Fentanyl transdermal patches for Mom to decrease her pain. In addition to the therapies Mom was receiving, I asked the DON if she knew any massage therapists who would come to the home to give Mom a weekly massage.

40

Small Comforts & Seven Stages

Lori and I knew that Medicaid insurance would not cover massage therapy, though this is now a matter of debate and may vary by state Medicaid laws. After analyzing Mom's bank statements and monthly bills, we realized we had sufficient funds in the conservatorship account to cover massage therapy for at least a year. After that, I would use the account I had set aside for Mom.

Lori and I were on good terms again. I did not want any miscommunications about the money I had for Mom, so I transferred half of it into an account in Lori's name. I suggested she use it for Mom's necessities when the conservator account was low.

After we arranged the necessary funds, Lori and I began searching for a licensed massage therapist. Several staff members at the facility recommended Sharon. She was willing to come to the home and provide weekly massage sessions for Mom. She said these sessions would help ease the pain and stiffness of her contractures. I arranged a day and time for us to meet with her so she could assess Mom.

For the next three years, Sharon worked with Mom weekly. She never fully recovered much strength or muscle movement, but I believe she had less pain. Overall, her physical and mental condition had clearly deteriorated during the latter part of 1997 and throughout 1998. It was heartbreaking to watch.

It wasn't until the fall of 1998 that the administrator issued a thirty-day written notice of the facility's intent to transfer Mom to a room on the long-term care wing. By then, we were well-prepared for the transfer and had met with several of the staff who would be caring for Mom.

The term custodial care—also known as total care—is a component of long-term care. Staff sometimes use this term to refer to a long-term care resident who requires assistance with all daily activities, such as bathing, eating, dressing, and toileting.

Although I had seen it coming for a year, the realization that my mother was in the late stages of Alzheimer's disease was another assault on my heart. Knowing it would never get better, I had to remind myself that I could still do what was in my power to minimize her pain and discomfort. I had to repeat this to myself.

As we prepared for this last phase of the disease, we collaborated with the facility to ensure she received specialized care. We requested regular updates on any changes in her condition or comfort needs. It was of the utmost importance that Mom continue to receive passive range of motion exercises, frequent skin integrity checks, and daily routines such as applying moisturizer to her extremities. She also required specific positioning support and careful feeding to minimize the risk of aspiration.

Our goal was to provide maximum comfort. Just as important, we wanted to maintain her dignity throughout this continuing sorrowful journey.

Dr. Barry Reisberg, Director of the Fisher Alzheimer's Disease Education and Research Program at NYU Grossman School of Medicine, is recognized for identifying and developing "The Seven Stages of Alzheimer's." The stages may not always be clearly apparent in a person, and there is no definitive timeline for each period. However, these stages serve as a guide to caregivers in designing a care plan. Some people progress quickly through the disease and die within a few years after diagnosis. Others may live twenty years or more.

The Alzheimer's Association offers a document outlining the Seven Stages. This guide describes what one can expect in a specific stage. (See Resources for website.)

The Seven Stages, as identified by Reisberg, are:

Stage 1: No impairment
Stage 2: Very mild cognitive decline
Stage 3: Mild cognitive decline
Stage 4: Moderate cognitive decline
Stage 5: Moderate to severe cognitive decline
Stage 6: Severe cognitive decline
Stage 7: Very severe cognitive decline (final stage)

In stages one and two, a person may feel they are experiencing memory loss, though others usually do not notice any signs. However, as the condition progresses to stage three, loved ones may begin to observe the person's difficulties in finding the right words, losing items, or struggling to complete household chores and errands.

I recall that during these early periods, Mom would forget names or specific words mid-conversation. Sometimes, she would stop talking and look around with a blank stare. Initially, these episodes were few and far between, but they became more frequent and evident over time. As she progressed into stage three, we became more aware of these lapses. We observed her struggle to complete everyday tasks such as cleaning or making a meal, and frequently misplacing items—like the time she put the phone in the freezer.

During the middle and late stages, we observed Mom's increasing difficulty with conversation and recalling events. Specifically, she would increasingly forget what she wanted to say and stop talking mid-sentence. She began getting lost while driving to appointments and places she had frequented for years.

Her physical abilities changed as well. She began walking with hesitation, and her balance slowly declined until she needed a walker to ambulate. We also observed a slow decline in her ability to feed herself. During mealtime, she initially required gentle reminders to eat and use her utensils. Occasionally, she needed a hand to guide hers; but eventually, she needed a firm hand to help guide the food to her mouth.

During the seventh, or last stage of Alzheimer's, Mom required total care, including the management of incontinence of bowel and bladder. By this period, she rarely spoke and required complete support for daily activities. She was fed by the staff or one of her children during our visits. Although she rarely smiled anymore, there were moments during my visits when a glimmer of recognition would appear; her eyes would brighten as she looked into mine.

After over two years in memory care at Oakwood, Mom's move to their long-term care wing marked a new adjustment for us. Although the transition went smoothly for her, it clearly emphasized her downward trajectory to my siblings and me.

41

Mom Turns Sixty-Four

By winter 1999, Mom had settled into a room in Oakwood's newly completed long-term care unit. She had lived in two facilities, spending four years in memory care units before her legs betrayed her. Although medically stable, she was now totally dependent on the staff. She could sit in a recliner or wheelchair, or lie in bed, but she could no longer move on her own. Trained caregivers could transfer her using a Hoyer lift without risk of injury. This device, operated by a hydraulic pump, made moving Mom safe and easy. We were grateful for the caregivers who remained attentive to her positioning and comfort needs.

The atmosphere in the unit was quiet and calming. Mom rarely recognized anyone, but on occasion, she would surprise us with her recall. Every time I walked into her room, I approached her and said, "Hi, Mom." Then, I would kiss her cheek while embracing her and, in a cheerful voice say, "I love you, Mom." Sometimes, moisture filled her eyes and tears streamed down her cheeks. While gently dabbing her face dry, I would see a moment of recognition in her gaze. My face would form a bittersweet smile as I leaned in to kiss her forehead.

My heart ached for my mother. She was a grandmother, aunt, sister, friend, neighbor, and caregiver. She was still here with us, living imprisoned in a body that no longer treated her well. Her life had been cut short, and the unfairness of it pierced my soul.

Based on information in the medical records and our own observations, Lori wrote in the conservatorship "Personal Well-Being Report" for the period of March 1998 through March 1999: "Does not respond verbally—she does not eat on her own, walk at all, and is incontinent. She occasionally smiles and follows you with her eyes. More calm...off all neuroleptic medications at this time. Her aggressive emotional behavior has decreased."

On March 8, 1999, Mom turned sixty-four. I returned to St. Paul to honor her. We reserved the conference room, and my siblings and their families came to celebrate her birthday. We were committed to Mom's quality of life, so these gatherings gave us emotional nourishment as we tried to preserve her dignity and provide some joy in her life.

We brought food to share. My mom was on a mechanical soft diet, a type of texture-modified diet designed for individuals who have difficulty chewing or swallowing. Because she had always loved McDonald's fish sandwiches, we bought one and ground it up so it met the requirements of a mechanical soft meal. She also enjoyed Starbucks hazelnut lattes, so we brought one for her. We fed her small bites and gave her small sips, monitoring her ability to swallow.

Ironically, at about 130 pounds, Mom weighed more than ever, except perhaps during her pregnancies. Even though she was unable to feed herself, she ate everything we gave her. Her ability to swallow, which often hinders the eating process in people with advanced Alzheimer's, was not yet an issue on her prescribed diet. My siblings and I were pleased to see Mom enjoying her food. She had been conscious of her weight her whole life. Other than her pregnancies, I don't believe she ever weighed over 110 pounds for her five-foot frame.

Notwithstanding her decline, Mom was sitting up in her wheelchair at the head of the table in the family room at the facility. She seemed to enjoy her sentimental birthday party and even shared moments of recognition. Despite the difficult times, we laughed and joked, wanting to appreciate this time together.

*****

Nearly eighteen months had passed since I closed on my house in Albuquerque. I was happily settled in my neighborhood, enjoying the hiking trails nearby. While I loved living in New Mexico and made good friends, I missed my mom. Caregiver fatigue had become a normal part of my life, a constant pull between my professional commitments and the emotional weight of being far from my mom.

My job required travel to client nursing facilities nationwide. When traveling, I added a day or two to visit Minnesota. I continued to let Lori know when I was in town, but I didn't always have time to call or see my other siblings.

While Steve physically recovered from his brain injury, his short-term memory deficit made it difficult for him to manage on his own. He called me often in 1998 and 1999, sharing that he was going through a divorce. He confided that he was unable to handle his finances and asked if I would serve as his power of attorney and assist him with healthcare and medical decision-making. And, to my surprise, he asked if I would help him find a place to live. Consequently, my visits to Minnesota were usually extended to help him.

I enjoyed my job and continued to learn a great deal about the continuum of long-term care. However, it was difficult at times, balancing my personal experiences and providing legal advice to client nursing homes on some of the same issues I was dealing with as a daughter. The fortunate aspect was that working in the profession enriched my understanding of how to advocate for Mom in the maze of long-term care issues.

It worked both ways. As a lawyer, I helped my client administrators and nursing staff understand families' perspectives in a positive way. In facility disputes with family members, I was often able to help administrators or staff resolve issues through a collaborative approach.

The long-term care profession is vulnerable to litigious activity. Specifically, alleged malpractice or wrongful death lawsuits are common in the long-term care profession. Some situations are quite serious—involving accidents or significant mistakes—but others could have been resolved through astute communication and empathy.

Family members often threaten to sue a facility when they are angry about something that happened to their loved one. As a corporate operations attorney, I often received calls from administrators about issues that were not strictly legal concerns but, if left unaddressed, might escalate to legal action.

For instance, one administrator called me to say that a daughter wished to assist the facility in giving her mother a bath once a week in the late afternoon or evening. The facility informed her that they scheduled all residents' baths in the mornings, three days a week, and were unable to change the times. The daughter became angry and started raising other concerns, threatening to sue for a fall and subsequent injury her mother had sustained months earlier—an issue she had previously let go. I immediately thought about my mom— easily putting myself in the daughter's position. I spoke to the administrator and shared how important it might be for the daughter to feel she was contributing to her mother's care. The facility agreed to work with her.

A little communication and compromise on both sides goes a long way toward easing family and resident stress and smoothing tensions with the facility. It may ultimately prevent a claim or lawsuit. Reflecting on Mom's journey reminds me that it was the staff who were willing to both discuss issues with me and follow through on her care measures that gave me a sense of comfort and allowed me to let my guard down.

42

A Family Affair

Over the challenging years of long-distance caregiving, I spent time in reflection, wishing I could move my mom to a facility in Albuquerque to be closer to me. However, I knew it would be traumatic to transfer her to a new setting again, much less across the cultural chasm from Minnesota to New Mexico. I also knew that my siblings would not agree to such a move, so I never took action.

Sometimes, I believed it would have been easier to be an only child dealing with Mom's illness. My thoughts often vacillated between wishing I had sole responsibility for Mom and feeling grateful not to have to carry the burden alone. In reality, I knew I was fortunate to have my siblings. Even through tough times and difficult communications, it was ultimately better for Mom to have many people in her life who loved her. And it was better for me.

Family and close friends visited Mom regularly, including my Aunt Gussie and a few of my cousins. Mom seemed to recognize my aunt's voice and would occasionally turn to gaze at her with love in her eyes when my aunt sang, told stories, or shared sisterly gossip. Sparks of weathered memories continued to burn when my aunt visited. Mom had always admired her oldest sibling and sought her advice throughout her life. We were able to overcome the hard feelings between us that arose when my aunt initially took a firm stance against my siblings and me in the dispute with Rodney.

Gussie was gutsy, especially for women of her generation. She was a member of a singing group called "Millie and Her Dogpatch Dollies." As the mistress of ceremonies, she introduced the performers, but also had her star moments singing and dancing. The other women in the group played wash tubs and other homemade instruments while Millie played the piano. They performed at nursing homes, churches, and hospitals, never accepting monetary remuneration. They may have even played at the facility where Mom lived.

Mom had several close high school girlfriends whom she had always admired. While they didn't get together often over the years because they were raising families and didn't live nearby, she kept in touch and talked fondly of the good times they shared. When we received Christmas cards from them every year, Mom would regale me with stories of their friendship and confidences. When I was in high school, she encouraged me to work hard, but also to enjoy myself—sharing that those were some of her best years. She regretted leaving school in the fall of her senior year to follow Dad during his Army transfers. I was pleased to hear that these friends visited Mom.

Lori and her husband, John, visited regularly with their children. Lori worked as a home health aide and later as a certified nursing assistant. As an employee of the facility's sister home health business which had an office in Oakwood's building, she was able to look in on Mom when she went to the office.

Over time, as Lori's work strengthened her understanding of the importance of preventing contractures and skin sores, she would examine Mom during visits. She massaged Mom's arms and hands, ensuring her splints were clean and fit properly. She worked closely with the facility staff to ensure that Mom received adequate nutrition on a regular basis. And although weight loss is a concern in the Alzheimer's resident, there were times when Mom was gaining weight, and Lori would work with the staff to limit Mom's snacks or excess calories.

All of Mom's grandchildren brought her joy, always. And being in a nursing facility was no different. As Lori's daughter, Andrea, approached the age for a summer job, she began working in the kitchen at the nursing home, allowing her to visit her grandma every time she worked. And in keeping with Mom's love of music, Lori's son, Joey, played the trumpet; he performed at the facility during several holiday celebrations.

Living in close proximity to the facility, Dan and Lynn visited Mom frequently. They often arrived at dinner time to help feed her. As time allowed, Cheri and her husband would drive down from northern Minnesota for the day. Cheri told me they didn't often let others know they were in town because she wanted time alone with Mom. Usually, they could only get away for a day at a time.

Sissy and her husband, Brian, visited the facility often, and after February 1998, they brought their beautiful daughter—Mom's newest grandchild. After Brian's grandmother became a resident at Oakwood, Sissy's mother-in-law stopped by to see Mom when she visited her own mother.

When I was in town, Steve would often accompany me to the facility. While he never regained his short-term memory, he was able to live alone during this time period. As he requested, I helped him settle into a mobile home in Inver Grove Heights, which I had purchased on his behalf using an annuity he had retained after his divorce. I was grateful that he had a place of his own. Yet, the weight of responsibility was intense, knowing how much he depended on me.

He lived two doors down from the mobile home community manager. I spoke with her about his short-term memory loss, his coma, and his extensive rehabilitation. She agreed to keep on eye on him and contact me with any concerns. If she didn't see him working in his yard or coming and going for a few days, she would notify me.

Steve was reinstated to his job and had his driver's license renewed after a full physical recovery. However, he was soon relieved of his duties after the company realized that his short-term memory was an issue and that he could not adequately perform the roofing work for the school district. They advised him to sign up for Social Security disability. He also had to relinquish his driver's license within the year.

I helped Steve navigate community and veteran services to arrange rides to medical appointments or other destinations he wanted to visit. Some friends looked in on him. While a few were bad influences regarding his tendency to drink or smoke weed, others truly cared.

Mom would have been upset by Steve's permanent memory loss. For once, I counted her lack of awareness as a small blessing.

*****

As time passed, our confidence in the staff of the long-term care wing grew. To promote continuity of care, the facility did a good job of assigning the same certified nursing assistant to each resident when possible. When Mom moved to the unit in the fall of 1998, we hung another memory board with pictures of all of us and the grandchildren. Although Mom's recognition of others decreased over time, we knew that her long-term memory was the last to fade, so we included pictures of her mother, siblings, and high school friends.

We did this for several reasons. First, we wanted to be prompted by the pictures so we could talk to Mom, recount the stories she told, and share our own memories with her. Also, we wanted the staff to know that Mom had had a life full of family and friends before her disease robbed her of the ability to share her own stories. Many of the staff members asked questions and showed genuine interest in their residents' and families' photos, recognizing these pictures as valuable windows into the individual lives of the residents they cared for on a daily basis.

Connie, a certified nursing assistant assigned to Mom several days a week, was looking at the photos one day when Lori was present. She pointed to a picture on the bulletin board next to Mom's bed and asked if she could take it home for the evening and show it to her dad. She believed it was his high school picture. She asked Lori if she could share my mom's name and condition with her dad to confirm if he knew her. Lori agreed.

The next day, Connie brought the picture back, confirming it was her dad in the photo. She shared that her dad had dated Mom briefly in high school and wanted to visit her, which was okay with us. Sadly, Mom didn't show any signs of recognition when he arrived for a visit—he expected this, given what his daughter had told him.

Nonetheless, he took the time to talk to her, sharing his sadness that she had to go through so much suffering.

I was grateful for all of Mom's visitors. We never knew what she might hear, or when she would have flashes of clarity. She was still with us, and occasional moments of recognition made our day. In those uncertain times, we clung to the moments of noticeable recall that she still had hidden within her.

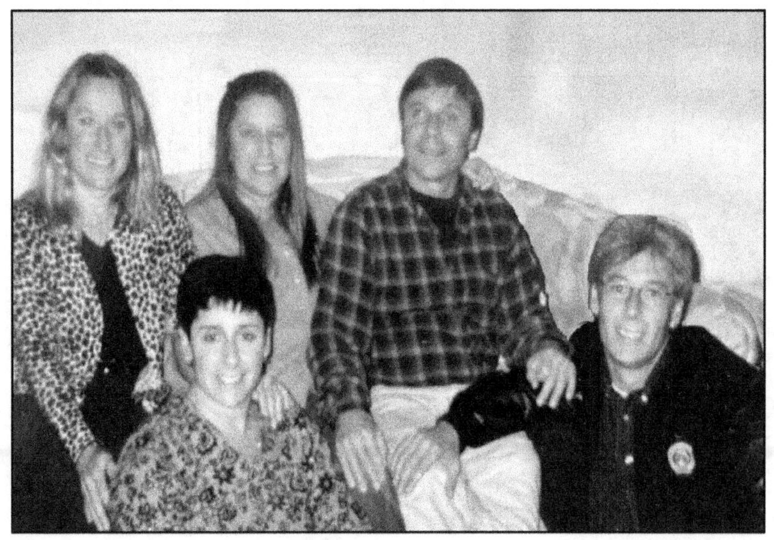

Siblings: Kathleen, Cheri, Steve, Lori, and Dan

43

Looking for Blessings

L ooking for small blessings as Mom's mind and body withered in the last stages of Alzheimer's—yet remained stable medically—was difficult, but I found a few.

In 1999, she had no acute illnesses. She ate most meals when fed. If she lost weight, the facility would add Ensure supplements between meals to maintain a healthy weight. Totally dependent on the staff for all her care, she could not communicate her needs or wishes in any meaningful way. Her contractures were being managed with massage, splinting, and passive range of motion exercises, and pain medications continued to keep her comfortable.

During visits, I sat with Mom, shared memories, held and massaged her hands and arms, and played big band or country music. Occasionally, she responded to the sounds she loved, and I detected a slight sway in her body as she moved to the familiar rhythm. Although I did not know for certain what she heard or understood, I kept talking, hoping for a moment of recall. Most times, I did not know what I said that triggered the moment, but there it was: her eyes opened wide, her face relaxed, and a slight smile emerged. A small blessing.

My faith in God comforted me. Although I had not attended church regularly for years, I began attending again after moving to Albuquerque. I prayed. I prayed for Mom, my siblings, their families, and myself. I prayed for continued strength in helping Mom get through the Alzheimer's disease process without pain. Finally, I prayed that my trips to Minnesota would allow me to simply be a daughter visiting her mother, not a nurse, lawyer, or conservator.

Gradually, I began to feel at peace with my mom, sitting and chatting simply as her daughter. This peace felt like a direct response to my prayers, marking a shift from my earlier stress and conflict. As I relaxed, the conflicts about her care, my own mental strife, and family disagreements gradually decreased.

Still, the emotional pain continued to stab at my heart. I hated to see Mom so incapable of enjoying life, seemingly oblivious to her environment and anyone around her. Year after year, nothing changed, and my earlier sense of peace gave way to anger. Why is she still here? What purpose does it serve God for Mom to live like this? I began to pray for an end to her suffering. Some say that early-onset Alzheimer's runs a faster course, but that was not our experience.

I prayed: *Please God, take my mom. She is ready to be with You. We are ready. I begged Him; I questioned Him. Why are You keeping her here on earth? She would not have wanted to be dependent on others all these years. Please, if there is no hope of recovery, take her so she can be with our dad, our grandmother Helene, and her sister, Betty, in heaven.*

*****

Amid these personal challenges, a significant shift occurred in my professional life. My career took a turn in the spring of 1999 when I was laid off from my job as Corporate Counsel for Sun Healthcare Group because the corporation filed for bankruptcy. It was a shock. I had been in Albuquerque less than two years, had taken another state bar exam, and bought a lovely house. I thought I would be in New Mexico for a long time.

Though I received job offers, I did not want to relocate again. The long-term care industry was turbulent during this period—with frequent company acquisitions and restructuring. After taking three different state bar examinations, I decided not to risk relocation for another job that might require me to take yet another test.

I took classes on starting a business, specifically a law practice. I networked with Albuquerque lawyers and sought their advice on starting a small healthcare law practice. After conducting extensive research and networking, I opened a law firm and consulting practice in 1999 specializing in representing healthcare providers.

Transitioning into self-employment, I continued to work with long-term care facilities while also reaching out to risk management companies. I evaluated risk in long-term care entities for liability insurance purposes. Having my own business meant I had to be ever vigilant in securing and retaining clients. As business grew, I worked long hours and spoke at state and national conferences. My clients included local facilities, regional companies, and national clients who owned long-term care entities in New Mexico.

Traveling for work gave me the flexibility to return to Minnesota to see my mom and to assist Steve. Despite having more control over my work, feelings of exhaustion crept into my life, but I tried to ignore them. I was tired and weary. My energy levels were depleted. While prayer gave me comfort and focus, I did not see any miracle. However, I observed stability and consistency in Mom's care.

We entered 2000 without the devastating Y2K fanfare that the world had anticipated. 2000 passed. And so did 2001. Mom remained medically stable in late-stage Alzheimer's disease.

As the new millennium unfolded, my family responsibilities grew. Helping Steve was demanding, especially in the spring of 2002, when he fell into another coma for a few weeks. He was a patient in the Veterans Hospital in Minneapolis for two months, requiring me—as his attorney-in-fact and healthcare agent—to be intensely involved in his care issues. I traveled to Minnesota to attend several of his care conferences and to plan for his discharge to a nursing facility for another two months, after which he returned to his home. Of course, I would visit Mom too. I knew she would be comforted that I was watching out for Steve.

Despite juggling family and work, I found unexpected moments of connection. One day, while I was sitting at my desk writing a legal report, the mother of a dear high school friend called. She was visiting Albuquerque with her husband, Tom. I knew and loved her, often visiting her at home when I was in St. Paul. During a delightful lunch, as I listened to stories about their travels, Mary turned to me and asked about my life, my mom, and my brother. I shared the most recent updates. She exclaimed, "No wonder you aren't married. You don't have time!" While I did not see this as the reason I wasn't married, her comment gave me pause for reflection.

Contemplating Mary's comments, I realized how unpredictable life is. We do what is required to take care of our family and loved ones. Our lives may be interrupted, placing us on unexpected paths, but we can accept these changes as part of life. Life's turns shape us as we navigate rough roads. I believe new beginnings are always around the corner if we embrace flexibility and resilience.

Part VI

Resolution and Reconciliation

Kathleen A. Hessler

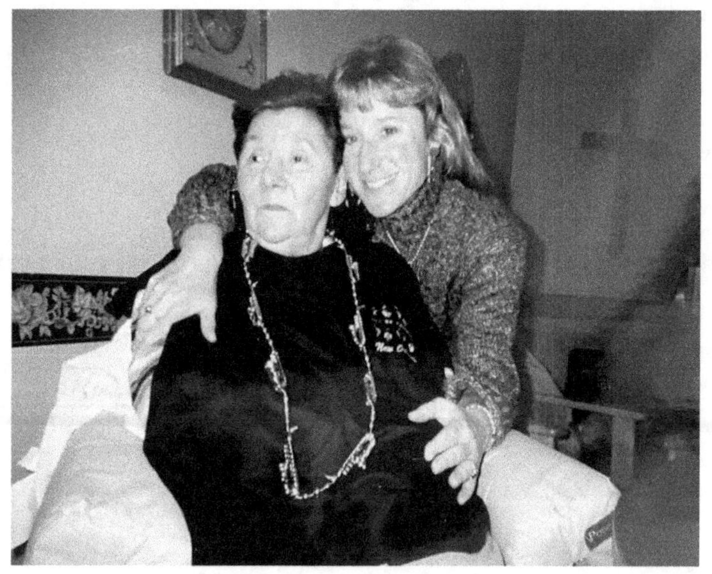

Mom and Kathleen at Oakwood Nursing Facility

44

Treasures of Long-Term Care

My boutique law and consulting practice thrived for over a decade. Managing my own business gave me control over my schedule, which was crucial as I navigated ongoing care issues with my mom and Steve.

My primary clients were national long-term care companies that retained me as counsel for state and federal regulatory appeals, specifically when providers received deficiencies during mandatory Medicare surveys. Additionally, I served as their local counsel, conducting investigations and providing legal guidance on complex regulatory and risk management issues.

For regional and local companies, I functioned as an outsourced general counsel, risk manager, and compliance executive. These relationships were typically structured on a retainer basis, ensuring a consistent monthly commitment. Beyond my core legal work, I specialized in healthcare ethics, serving on bioethics committees for several organizations.

I successfully minimized overhead by establishing a home-based office long before it became an accepted professional practice. Because my clients typically preferred on-site consultation, I structured my time for maximum productivity. I dedicated mornings to writing and research, taking advantage of the early hours to draft legal arguments for my client cases. My afternoons were devoted to more interactive tasks, such as telephone interviews or visiting client buildings, providing staff education, and investigating accidents or unexpected incidents.

In addition to my day-to-day work, speaking around the country at legal and healthcare conferences provided new opportunities for networking and brainstorming with colleagues. We discussed important long-term care legal and ethical issues encountered daily. This information became invaluable in understanding and working with Oakwood as well as supporting Mom and Steve.

One particular opportunity grew out of these professional connections. The national company that owned Oakwood, also operated several entities in New Mexico. Their general counsel, whom I met at a conference, hired me to represent them in legal actions at their New Mexico locations. I bonded quickly with their staff after sharing that my mother lived in one of their homes in Minnesota. This gave me a unique perspective on the company's values and operations, which helped me appreciate the care my mom received daily, even as we navigated some challenges.

The nurses, aides, doctors, therapists, social workers, administrators, dietary personnel, activities staff, and housekeeping and maintenance employees I met during my career inspired confidence in the long-term care profession. Many direct caregivers do this work out of a genuine passion for helping people. They work tirelessly, demonstrating compassion and skill by taking an interest in learning about their residents and families. When homes are short-staffed, these dedicated workers often take on double shifts.

In August 2002, I had the opportunity to speak at the New Mexico Healthcare Association (NMHCA) conference, the trade association for nursing facilities in New Mexico. I was hired by them on several occasions to represent NMHCA at hearings in Santa Fe when new state regulations were proposed. The Association organizes several educational conferences each year for nursing home executives and staff. Fun activities provide a space for the attendees to relax, learn, and exchange information. I was a frequent speaker at these conferences and an enthusiastic supporter of their hard work. I provided personal examples of my experiences with my mom during my presentations.

After speaking at the August 2002 conference themed "*Discover the Treasures of Long-Term Care*," I wrote a letter of thanks to the Association's members. The letter was published in their fall newsletter that year. As I wrote the letter, I recalled the laughter and heartfelt speeches during the awards luncheon. I typed: "I wish to thank each and every one of you who continue to dedicate yourselves and give your best in this increasingly complex and demanding environment..."

I grew to appreciate and respect the people working in this emotionally and physically challenging profession. What I wrote back then still stands today: "I speak from personal experience when I say your sincerity in getting to know your families and residents goes a long way in warming the hearts of family members, especially when the resident isn't aptly able to express...the essence of their person." I referenced the CNA, Connie, who studied my mom's photos and identified her dad as someone my mom dated in high school.

I wrote not only about the challenging issues in the industry, but also about the heartwarming moments my family and I shared with the staff at the facility where Mom resided. I spoke about the importance of maintaining a sense of humor and the many kindnesses we received.

Many in this profession, especially direct caregivers, may not acquire great material wealth; however, their empathy, gentleness, and physical labor exemplify their humanity, enriching the lives of both residents and families. I closed my letter expressing deep appreciation for these professionals, hoping they continue to find inspiration in the 'small treasures' of gratitude they receive.

Kathleen A. Hessler

45

The End of Suffering

The final, or seventh stage, of Alzheimer's disease can last anywhere from a few weeks to several years. Mom's course was the latter. Although she was unable to initiate any interaction, I believed she could still hear and enjoy music. And I know she benefited from gentle touch, as do all human beings.

When I visited, I would play her favorite music. I also read old letters and magazine articles to her, and showed her photos of family and friends. Sometimes, when listening to some of her favorite tunes, I would look into her eyes, lean in, and whisper: "Mom, remember how you loved to move to the rhythm of this song when you made dinner in the kitchen?" I hoped to kindle a comforting memory for her.

Her skin was dry, and it felt good to apply soothing lotion to her arms and legs while gently massaging them. If the weather was sunny and warm, I would push the wheelchair outside to one of the patios at the facility.

In late-stage Alzheimer's, monitoring a person's capability to eat becomes critical. When fed, Mom would open her mouth and accept the food, but her ability to chew decreased over time. Sometimes, with prompting, she would continue to eat or move the food around in her mouth for a few minutes, but then stop. Because of this, the person feeding her had to remain vigilant to ensure she did not aspirate.

In other words, it was critical to prevent food from bypassing the esophagus and being sucked into the airway, a process called aspiration. When food or liquid unintentionally enters and settles in the lungs, it can cause aspiration pneumonia, a medical condition characterized by infection and inflammation. This problem is common during the final stages of Alzheimer's disease.

Mom's first episode occurred in early fall of 2002. The facility called to inform me that she was diagnosed with aspiration pneumonia. Since her advance directives stated she did not want life-prolonging measures, they asked if they should treat the bacterial pneumonia with antibiotics. Knowing that pneumonia can be painful, and that oral antibiotics can increase comfort by decreasing fever and other symptoms—even when death is imminent—Lori and I consented.

But, deep inside, I grappled with a quiet unease. Would this decision truly bring her relief, or were we prolonging her suffering? Mom's nurses were able to give her the medication with small amounts of pureed food. Her pneumonia was cured, but she had a recurrence within a couple of weeks. We opted for the same course of treatment, hoping it was the right choice amid the inevitable outcome.

The third occurrence of pneumonia was in mid-November 2002. At that time, the medical director advised us that another course of oral antibiotics was prohibitive because Mom had virtually stopped taking anything by mouth. The only option for treating the pneumonia was with intravenous antibiotics, which involved delivering medication directly into the vein. Lori and I knew this would cause more pain and discomfort to Mom and prolong her suffering.

In keeping with her advance directives, we did not agree to intravenous treatment. Rather, we agreed to symptomatic comfort measures, providing oxygen, pain medications (fentanyl patch), and frequent repositioning. Additionally, the staff and our family provided other end-of-life care measures, such as skin exams, massage with moisturizer, PROM exercises, and other comfort measures, including consistent mouth care using moisturized swabs.

In 2002, unlike today, hospice was not a common consideration for people with Alzheimer's disease. Looking back, it is important to recognize that when the Medicare hospice benefit was initiated in 1983 for end-of-life care, the focus was on care for patients with cancer. Over the years, hospice enrollment has evolved to include patients with end-stage heart disease, pulmonary disease, and many other non-cancer diagnoses, such as Alzheimer's.

Medicare and many insurance companies will pay for hospice care in a patient's home (which includes residents who live in nursing homes). Hospice provides intermittent end-of-life care through scheduled visits from a team of hospice nurses, aides, social workers, and chaplains—with oversight by the hospice physician. If the patient has a need for high-level pain management with injections or a morphine drip, the patient may receive round-the-clock nursing care for several days at home, or they may receive care at a hospice inpatient unit.

Hospice is not just for the patient. It focuses on the family's well-being. Often, hospice workers train family members to perform care measures to ease the patient's discomfort. Looking back, I think admitting Mom to hospice care the last several months of her life would have been a benefit to all of us. Today, many families elect hospice for their loved ones who have end-stage Alzheimer's.

I knew death was close for Mom. She would not be able to overcome the pneumonia. Her advance directives essentially prohibited the placement of a feeding tube because it would prolong her life. Today, it is widely recognized that feeding tubes in patients with progressive Alzheimer's disease are futile and are not generally offered as an option by the medical staff. However, there may be exceptional cases where a healthcare provider believes a feeding tube would benefit a patient.

Lori and I had been in close contact during Mom's episodes of aspiration pneumonia and treatments thereof, especially the last episode when she received palliative care only. Because it was difficult to know when the exact time would come, I did not travel back to Minnesota to wait with her.

Those present at Mom's bedside when she passed were Lori, Dan, his wife, and daughter, and my sister Cheri. When I received the call from Lori, I was not shocked. I expected it. While I had said everything I wanted to say to Mom, I still experienced mixed feelings of guilt and sadness because I was not there at the end. Yet, knowing she was finally released from her daily struggles, I felt a peace I had not realized in a long time.

At sixty-seven, Mom took her last breath in this world on November 21, 2002. She was one of the approximately thirty percent of people with Alzheimer's who die of aspiration pneumonia as a result of the severity of their disease.

When I heard Mom had passed, I made arrangements immediately to fly to Minnesota. Mom was at peace. I felt relieved and happy for her that she could move on to heaven. I could visualize her there, whole and at peace. She had been given the final gift of grace.

46

The Service and Sentiments

While traveling to St. Paul for my mom's service in November 2002, I thought about her story of returning from Colorado for her own mother's funeral. Mom was only eighteen; my grandmother's death was sudden and unexpected. Mom was conflicted as to whether she should make the trip. In the end, she did, and the gathering of her siblings to mourn the loss of her mother helped ease her devastation.

Unlike my grandmother's sudden death, my mom's passing was long-expected—a bittersweet blessing after years of sorrow. It was time. It was past time, but it was on God's time. Like my mom, I found comfort in having my siblings together to honor our mother and to say our last goodbyes. The days leading up to the service allowed for reflection and unity, helping to shape our shared grief into moments of connection.

At her service, I spoke and shared some of the stories in this book. I tried to convey the core of my mom's spirit, the gentleness of her soul. Many in attendance nodded as I spoke, affirming the memories we had collectively.

Although I sought closure, hoping only good memories would remain, the path to that point was not easy. For a long time, the sad recollections of her decline overshadowed the fond memories of her love, strength, and laughter. In writing this book, I realized that much of my story centers on my mom as a patient navigating an illness that consumed many years. I wanted others to know her beauty and ability to love and nurture. I wanted her essence to shine through, despite the ravages of the disease.

Notwithstanding death being long in coming, the feelings of loss were present with the finality of it all. The unrealized tension and stress of watching her edge into an inner world I could not reach built up over the years. Did I do all I could for her? Would she be proud of her children for the care we provided? Did she know how much she was loved? These had been ever-present questions—some laid to rest. For weeks after her death, I felt drained and raw. It was finally over.

Losing one's mother can be among life's most difficult challenges. The loss of a parent who offered so much love and influence is like losing a part of yourself. Although the mom I knew disappeared years before her death—because of the tragic reality of Alzheimer's—she was always my mom.

Toward the end, she was a mere shell of herself. Yet, when I looked into her blank eyes, I remembered the love we shared. I would say, "Mom, I love you." Occasionally, a tear rolled down her cheek. I would wipe it with a soft tissue and hug her close. "I know you are still here, Mom. I will never forget you, but you are free to go. Go be with Dad, with your mom," I would whisper. She finally did.

*****

Fortunately, we had little stress in dealing with the funeral home and services. In 1995, I had purchased a prepaid funeral package. The casket and other details were arranged in advance, which saved the stress of making last-minute decisions. We called the funeral home to inform them that Mom had passed. Funds remaining in the accounts that Lori and I held on behalf of Mom were divided equally and disbursed to my siblings after all arrangements were complete.

The service was performed at Saint Stanislaus church, the same Catholic church where Dad received his send-off. The same priest who directed Dad's funeral, beloved Father Clay, presided over Mom's service. She was laid to rest at Fort Snelling National Cemetery, next to Dad, after a touching burial ceremony in the cool November weather.

My siblings and I had dinner one night, sharing stories and tears. We were gentle with each other as we processed the loss of our mom.

I believed our past disagreements, arguments, and ill feelings, rooted in so much accumulated stress over the years, were finally laid to rest with Mom. At least for me, they were. Grace and forgiveness can heal past wounds when we give and accept these gifts. Holding on to resentments and anger breeds more stress and unhappiness in life.

Mom was an adoring and nurturing mother, a fun grandmother to eleven children, a caring auntie to many, a devoted home health aide to her clients, a loving caregiver to family members, and a loyal confidante to friends. She was known as Adele, but some people called her Dale. She is still my dear, sweet mother, and she will always be remembered and loved forever.

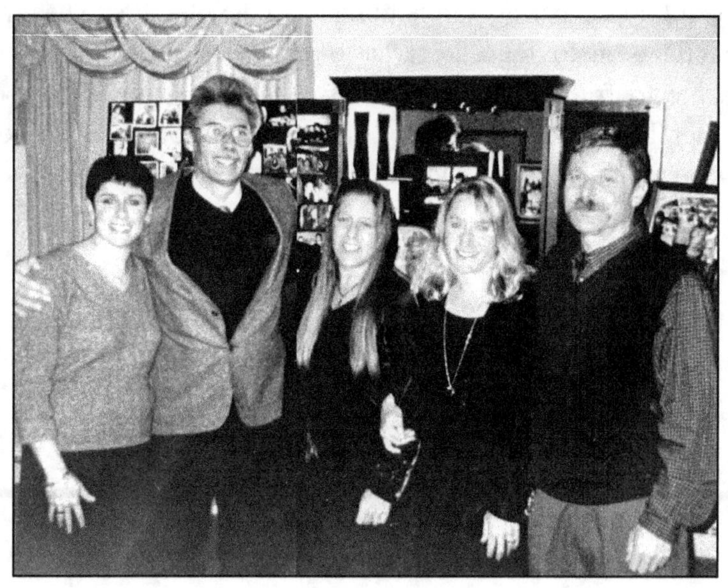

Lori, Dan, Cheri, Kathleen, and Steve at Mom's funeral

47

Mother's Day 2024

Mother's Day, twenty-two years after Mom died: I stand at my parents' gravesites in Fort Snelling National Cemetery, Minneapolis, Minnesota. Over the years, I have driven by the cemetery many times as I come and go from the airport. It is less than two miles from the terminal I fly into most often. Each time, I think of my parents, interred there. I recall my dad's burial on a cold, crisp January day in 1987, the ground frozen but almost bare of snow—and my mom's service in November 2002, a cool late-autumn day.

As I come to see family this May and pass by the National Cemetery on my way out of the airport, I wonder why I haven't been back to the beautiful grounds since Mom's burial. Why do I feel a strong urge to visit them this year? It is a tug I have never felt before. I hold no guilt; honoring gravesites was never my tradition. But why not?

I always thought Mom and Dad's souls had escaped the confines of their coffins and rose to the Grandest Place in the Sky. My dad's presence is strongest when I am out on a lake or enjoying the outdoors. It was during these times that I experienced the most peace with him. I think of him whenever I pass a Texaco station. Certain sayings of his resonate with me. I hear his voice: "It's a jungle out there, Kath." Or, "There is nothing free in this world…you have to work hard."

My mom is often on my mind when I create one of her original recipes, ride my bike, or admire the beauty of a garden. Eating fresh tomatoes reminds me of her garden, which she tended to every year. Traveling also brings her to mind. I know she would have treasured

265

the adventures it offers, if given the opportunity. I reflect on Mom's gentle spirit as I reread her old letters and stories, look through weathered photos, or gaze upon her early childhood art.

While finishing my book, I sifted through old boxes filled with important papers, photos, and other memories of my mom and our family. I found a few precious pieces of her childhood art. She enjoyed writing poems and stories. I discovered holiday poems she wrote in the third grade, along with her fourth-grade drawings and tales of other countries, written in 1944. Even as a child, Mom showed talent in writing and demonstrated her love of adventure.

The brown paper is crumpling, and the words are fading from pen and pencil. Pictures colored with crayons still show the brightness of their original reds, oranges, and greens. Her spirit shines through them. I cherish these drawings and reread the stories. My review of the tales she wrote at ten years old, along with the maps and pictures she drew, showed that Mom excelled in geography.

*****

Even though I feel my parents' presence in many ways, I suddenly felt a strong urge to visit the cemetery. During a visit with my brother Dan and his wife, Lynn, on the Saturday before I was scheduled to leave, I asked him if he had ever visited Mom and Dad's gravesites. "Why, yes, of course. Lynn and I visit several times a year," he said. His response was instantaneous.

I told him I had never returned. Surprised, he listened as I explained that it had been on my mind all week. Dan encouraged me. He described the flat gravestones, situated amidst the grassy part of the cemetery where our parents are buried, in contrast to the tall, white, and gray grave markers on most of the grounds. He texted me a photo of their gravesites and directions to section H.

The next day, around noon, before my flight, I entered the cemetery after waiting in a long line of cars. I suspected it was busier than most Sundays because it was Mother's Day. I drove around the grounds briefly to become acclimated. I took a few deep breaths as I stopped at one of the maps, then I drove to the location.

The sun paraded slowly across the brilliant blue sky, which was sprinkled with thin layers of white clouds. I stepped onto the bright green grass, glistening in the spring sun, and meandered between rows of headstones. The soft wind beckoned me to move with purpose, breathe the fresh air, and saunter among the people who rested with Mom and Dad. I suddenly felt free, as if I were unraveling old internal yarns and letting go of the past once and for all. A wave of relief washed over me; the moment was unexpected, yet deeply reassuring.

Feeling more confident, I walked up and down several rows, scanning the names on the gravestones. However, I could not find my parents' sites—there were far more flat markers than I had expected. *How will I find them in this large, sprawling field?* I wondered.

I called Dan. "Hi, Kath," he said. When I asked how to locate the headstones, Dan reminded me that the plot numbers were on the upper right-hand side of the stone. We both looked at the text and picture he had sent me on Saturday. The numbers were there—perhaps I had been too uneasy about my visit to pay attention to details. Dan stayed on the phone, talking as I wove through the rows of flat headstones until I spotted their names.

"I found them, Dan!" I said.

"Oh, good, Kath. I'm so glad. Sometimes when we go for a visit, we take flowers and set them on the headstone."

I looked up as he said this and saw a sprinkling of flower vases on gravesites around me. Bright colors popped from the long stretches of rich, green grass. I knelt down at Mom's site. Unexpectedly, I cried softly. He heard me.

"Kath," Dan said. "I'll let you go, so you can visit with them."

"Okay, Dan. Thanks so much for encouraging me to visit," I whispered into the phone before I hung up.

With muffled cries, I told Mom how much I missed her and that she would always hold a large space in my heart, and that I wrote a book about her life and love, her happiness and sadness. I wanted the world to know and love her like I do.

Surprised by my own emotion, I was thankful to be alone. It gave me time with Mom and Dad. I told them I had just visited Steve, who now lives in a healthcare center within a senior living community in southern Minnesota. After many years of living with Sissy and her family, he is doing well—meeting new people and engaging in activities like gardening, craft classes, bingo, and Bible study. The staff says he is a "bright light" in the home. Although he never regained his short-term memory, he communicates effectively and expresses his wishes.

As I said goodbye, I wished my mom a happy Mother's Day. Standing and kneeling at my parents' graves brought back fond memories and confirmed they are resting in peace. Driving away, I embraced the emotion of seeing their headstones and talking to them. I plan to return to visit again someday.

This visit reminded me of the values they passed on. In raising their six children, both Mom and Dad instilled in each of us the importance of kindness and a generous spirit. While we still navigate sibling disagreements and may not speak for longer periods than I would like, we eventually forgive one another and come together to cherish precious time.

In sharing memories, we add pieces to our own life's jigsaw puzzle. By listening to each other in earnest and without judgment, we can access missing memories—pieces that may now fit together more tightly. Some issues that were unresolved long ago may have dissipated with the passage of time; unsaid apologies have been accepted, and forgiveness has been extended. Each of our recollections may differ, but together, we create a richer, more complete picture of our lives.

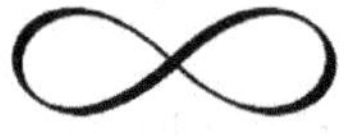

After Mom's death, in November 2002, my brother Dan wrote a heartfelt poem. I read it often because it brings me comfort.

"My Mom" by Dan J. Hessler

My Mother, Dale, well her time is done;
Now she's in heaven and having the fun.
Singing and dancing with my dear old Dad,
We'll miss you so much, oh how we're so sad.

She married so young to a guy known as Ray.
Love filled the house so all was O.K.
Mom worked so hard, she cooked and she cleaned;
She never ever slept—or at least so it seemed.
Her endless devotion to us and to Ray,
How could she do it each and every day?

When Ray left our lives, Mom was so torn;
She tried to move on even though so forlorn.
Mom and her dog, Penny, and all the Grandkids;
Some wine on occasion and enjoying her cigs…

Life was just fine with the love still around,
Until one day in her car, the house was not found.
Something was wrong with my dear mother;
An illness would take her, one like no other.
My siblings and I did research this disease;
We were torn up and angry, it brought Mom to her knees.

Up to the end she fought the good fight,
It soon to steal her, like a thief in the night.
Our loss here on earth is our Lord's gain.
Oh, my Dear God, please help with the pain.

We say good-byes in our own special ways,
To Mom, to Dale, now, together with Ray.

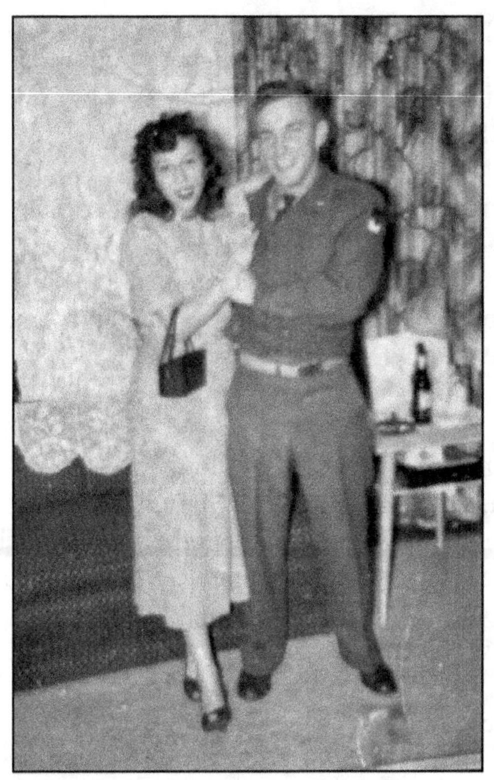

Adele and Ray circa 1952

Resources

- Alzheimer's Association: https://www.alz.org; Seven Stages of Alzheimer's Disease:

- National Institute on Aging: www.nia.nih.gov/alzheimers-disease-fact-sheet

- National Institute of Aging/Advance Directives: https://www.nia.nih.gov/health/advance-care-planning-advance-directives-health-care

- Dementia.org Healthcare Brands: www.dementia.org/stages-of-dementia

- Centers for Medicare and Medicaid: https://www.cms.gov

- Social Security: https://www.ssa.gov

Acknowledgments

First, I would like to thank Lori, my sister and friend, who shared conservator responsibilities with me in caring for our sweet mother. A heartfelt thank you to Lori's husband, John, who was a godsend in helping in many ways. Thank you also to all my siblings—Cheri, Steve, Dan, Lori, and Sissy—and their spouses, who contributed to Mom's care and quality of life in ways I may never know, because I was not always there. That would be their story.

I am grateful to all my siblings for taking my calls and responding to my texts. You helped refresh my memory as I worked on this manuscript over the years. I owe a debt of gratitude to my brother Dan, my sister Lori, and her husband, John. They reviewed my manuscript and provided honest, sometimes difficult, feedback. Thank you to my brother Steve, who listened as I read him chapters from the book. He confirmed he wanted me to tell his story too.

Dan, my brother, I appreciate the heartfelt poem you wrote about our mother, and I am grateful that you gave me permission to print it in this book.

Next, I would like to thank all my writing critique groups for providing sage advice through the years. Omar and Penny Durant, Margaret Tessler, Carol Kreis, and Kelly D. Williams reviewed my early draft. They encouraged me to delve further into my feelings, cut legalese, and speak simply—advice I truly tried to follow.

I am also grateful to my good friend Sherri L. Burr, who welcomed me into her critique group as a new member. That group, included author Judith Schiess Avila and physician Sue Brown. Their sincere advice helped me gain perspective and reframe issues. Their encouragement inspired me to open up and express my emotions as I told my story. Thank you for your insights and for sharing your truths.

I am grateful to all my beta readers and friends: Nancy Coleman, Diane Hoelzer, Helen Lechner, and Jo Ellen Siddens. Their honest opinions and continued encouragement gave me the confidence to share my book.

A heartfelt thank you to Sheree Bykofsky of Bykofsky and Associates, who read this book and encouraged me to pursue publishing it, providing valuable insights.

My gratitude and praise to Rose Kern of RMK Publications. She worked tirelessly on my behalf to format and publish this manuscript, and she also contributed her creative artwork to the cover.

A big thank you to Rosa B. Armijo-Pemble (imagesbyRosa.zenfolio.com) for my back-cover portrait. Her professional and creative work is accomplished with a personal touch that is unique to each of her clients.

I am endlessly grateful for my husband, Jim, whose patience, kindness, and encouragement have been a constant source of strength for me.

Finally, thank you to all the readers. Without you, I would not have written it. If you are a caregiver, I hope the stories inspired comfort, courage, and confidence. I hope they also provided information. You are not alone in navigating caregiving for a loved one. May you find healing and encouragement in your journey.

*****

I appreciate comments you may have about my book. Please consider leaving a review on the book's page on Amazon.com.

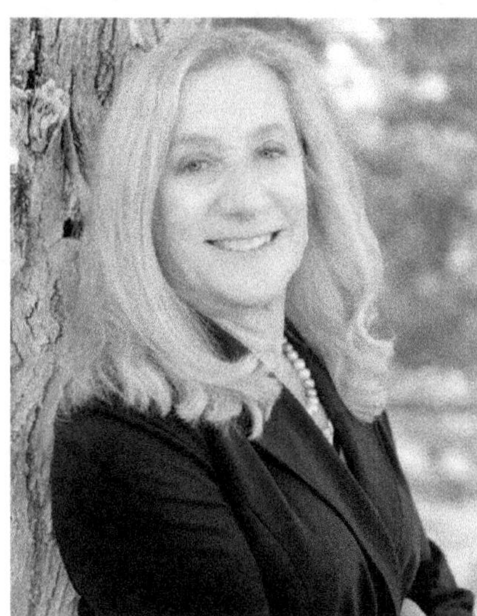

About the Author

Kathleen A. Hessler is an attorney and registered nurse with expertise in healthcare ethics and compliance. Her combined professions spanned several decades. During her nursing career, she provided direct patient care, conducted research, and managed teams. As an attorney and consultant, she guided long-term care facilities and other healthcare organizations through complex regulatory challenges. Her expertise has earned her recognition as a speaker at national healthcare and legal conferences.

She is a strong advocate for ethical patient care and sound business practices, bringing her unique perspective to nonfiction writing, which is her new focus. She contributed chapters for the *Solo Practice Guidebook* by The American Association of Nurse Attorneys (2025) and "Health Care Law" to the 2020 and 2024 editions of Giddens' *Concepts for Nursing Practice*. In addition to her professional writing, her award-winning nonfiction stories appear in SouthWest Writers anthologies.

When not at her computer, Kathleen enjoys reading, hiking scenic trails, playing golf, and traveling to new destinations with her husband.